Fat Grafting: Current Concept, Clinical Application, and Regenerative Potential, Part 1

Editors

LEE L.Q. PU
KOTARO YOSHIMURA
SYDNEY R. COLEMAN

CLINICS IN PLASTIC SURGERY

www.plasticsurgery.theclinics.com

April 2015 • Volume 42 • Number 2

ELSEVIER

1600 John F. Kennedy Boulevard • Suite 1800 • Philadelphia, Pennsylvania, 19103-2899

http://www.theclinics.com

CLINICS IN PLASTIC SURGERY Volume 42, Number 2
April 2015 ISSN 0094-1298, ISBN-13: 978-0-323-35983-2

Editor: Joanne Husovski
Developmental Editor: Donald Mumford

Clinics in Plastic Surgery (ISSN 0094-1298) is published quarterly by Elsevier Inc., 360 Park Avenue South, New York, NY 10010-1710. Months of issue are January, April, July, and October. Business and Editorial Offices: 1600 John F. Kennedy Blvd., Suite 1800, Philadelphia, PA 19103-2899. Periodicals postage paid at New York, NY and additional mailing offices. Subscription prices are $490.00 per year for US individuals, $716.00 per year for US institutions, $240.00 per year for US students and residents, $555.00 per year for Canadian individuals, $853.00 per year for Canadian institutions, $630.00 per year for international individuals, $853.00 per year for international institutions, and $305.00 per year for Canadian and foreign students/residents. To receive student/resident rate, orders must be accompanied by name of affiliated institution, date of term, and the signature of program/residency coordinator on institution letterhead. Orders will be billed at individual rate until proof of status is received. Foreign air speed delivery is included in all Clinics subscription prices. All prices are subject to change without notice. POSTMASTER: Send address changes to Clinics in Plastic Surgery, Elsevier Health Sciences Division, Subscription Customer Service, 3251 Riverport Lane, Maryland Heights, MO 63043. Customer Service: 1-800-654-2452 (US and Canada). From outside of the United States and Canada, call 314-447-8871. Fax: 314-447-8029. E-mail: JournalsCustomerService-usa@elsevier.com (for print support); JournalsOnlineSupport-usa@elsevier.com (for online support).

Reprints. For copies of 100 or more of articles in this publication, please contact the Commercial Reprints Department, Elsevier Inc., 360 Park Avenue South, New York, New York 10010-1710. Tel.: +1-212-633-3874; Fax: +1-212-633-3820; E-mail: reprints@elsevier.com.

Clinics in Plastic Surgery is covered in Current Contents, EMBASE/Excerpta Medica, Science Citation Index, MEDLINE/PubMed (Index Medicus), ASCA, and ISI/BIOMED.

Contributors

EDITORS

LEE L.Q. PU, MD, PhD, FACS
Professor, Division of Plastic Surgery, University of California, Davis, Sacramento, California

KOTARO YOSHIMURA, MD
Associate Professor, Department of Plastic Surgery, School of Medicine, University of Tokyo, Bunkyo-Ku, Tokyo, Japan

SYDNEY R. COLEMAN, MD
Clinical Assistant Professor of Plastic Surgery, New York University, New York, New York; University of Pittsburgh, Pittsburgh, Pennsylvania

AUTHORS

SEVERIANO DOS-ANJOS VILABOA, PhD
Stem Center, Palma de Mallorca, Spain

DINO ELYASSNIA, MD
Marten Clinic of Plastic Surgery, San Francisco, California

DAYONG GAO, PhD
Professor, Department of Mechanical Engineering, University of Washington, Seattle, Washington

SAHIL K. KAPUR, MD
Division of Plastic and Reconstructive Surgery, University of Wisconsin, Madison, Wisconsin

ADAM J. KATZ, MD, FACS
Department of Surgery, University of Florida College of Medicine, Gainesville, Florida

SHINICHIRO KUNO, MD
Department of Plastic Surgery, School of Medicine, University of Tokyo, Bunkyo-Ku, Tokyo, Japan

JENG-YEE LIN, MD, PhD
Assistant Professor, Division of Plastic Surgery, Taipei University Hospital, Taipei, Taiwan

RAMON LLULL, MD, PhD
Stem Center, Palma de Mallorca, Spain

KACEY G. MARRA, PhD
Departments of Bioengineering and Plastic Surgery, McGowan Institute for Regenerative Medicine, University of Pittsburgh, Pittsburgh, Pennsylvania

TIMOTHY J. MARTEN, MD
Founder and Director, Marten Clinic of Plastic Surgery, San Francisco, California

TAKANOBU MASHIKO, MD
Department of Plastic Surgery, School of Medicine, University of Tokyo, Bunkyo-Ku, Tokyo, Japan

ISABELLA C. MAZZOLA, MD
Plastic Surgeon, Department of Otolaryngology, Fondazione Ospedale Maggiore Policlinico IRCCS, Milano, Italy

RICCARDO F. MAZZOLA, MD
Consultant Plastic Surgeon, Department of Clinical Sciences and Community Health, Fondazione Ospedale Maggiore Policlinico IRCCS, Milano, Italy

DANIELLE M. MINTEER, BS
Department of Bioengineering, University of Pittsburgh, Pittsburgh, Pennsylvania

MÔNICA SARTO PICCOLO, MD, MSc
Director, Pronto Socorro para Queimaduras, Goiânia, Goiás, Brazil

MARIA THEREZA SARTO PICCOLO, MD, PhD
Scientific Director, Pronto Socorro para Queimaduras, Goiânia, Goiás, Brazil

NELSON SARTO PICCOLO, MD
Chief, Division of Plastic Surgery, Pronto Socorro para Queimaduras, Goiânia, Goiás, Brazil

LEE L.Q. PU, MD, PhD, FACS
Professor, Division of Plastic Surgery, University of California, Davis, Sacramento, California

J. PETER RUBIN, MD
Departments of Bioengineering and Plastic Surgery, McGowan Institute for Regenerative Medicine, University of Pittsburgh, Pittsburgh, Pennsylvania

ZHIQUAN SHU, PhD
Postdoctoral Fellow, Department of Mechanical Engineering, University of Washington, Seattle, Washington

LUIZ S. TOLEDO, MD
Consultant Plastic Surgeon – Dubai, Medical Arts Clinic, Dubai London Clinic, Saudi-German Hospital, Jumeirah, Dubai, United Arab Emirates

CHUNMEI WANG, MD, PhD
Professor and Chair, Department of Plastic and Aesthetic Surgery, Dongguan Kanghua Hospital, Dongguan, Guangdong, China

KOTARO YOSHIMURA, MD
Associate Professor, Department of Plastic Surgery, School of Medicine, University of Tokyo, Bunkyo-Ku, Tokyo, Japan

Contents

Fat injection empirically started 100 year ago to correct contour deformities mainly on the face and breast. The German surgeon Eugene Hollaender (1867-1932) proposed a cocktail of human and ram fat, to avoid reabsorption. Nowadays, fat injection has evolved, and it ranks among the most popular procedures, for it provides the physician with a range of aesthetic and reconstructive clinical applications with regenerative effects on the surrounding tissues. New research from all over the world has demonstrated the role of adipose-derived stem cells, present in the adipose tissue, in the repair of damaged or missing tissues.

Adipose tissue is a valuable, exploitable, appealing source of regenerative cells that can be used for a variety of clinical challenges. This article reviews the history of the development of adipose-derived cell science, particularly in the context of tissue engineering and regenerative medicine. It describes some of the advancements made in the field, as well as highlighting challenges and obstacles.

This article discusses adipose-derived stem cell (ASC) biology, describes the current knowledge in the literature for the safety and regulation of ASCs, and provides a brief overview of the regenerative potential of ASCs. It is not an exhaustive listing of all available clinical studies or every study applying ASCs in tissue engineering and regenerative medicine, but is an objective commentary of these topics.

Autologous fat grafting has become an important procedure for volumization and revitalization, although clinical outcomes depend greatly on technique. It was revealed recently how grafted fat tissue survives, regenerates, or dies. Experimental results provided the underlying mechanism and clinical implications for therapeutic strategies to maximize the effects of fat grafting, minimize necrosis, and avoid oil cyst formation.

Aspirated fat contains unnecessary components such as water, oil, and blood cells. For better outcomes, tissue purification and condensation are useful, especially when injection volume to the recipient site is limited. Because aspirated fat is relatively poor in adipose-derived stem/stromal cells (ASCs), ASC condensation seems important for obtaining better regeneration and retention. Reducing tissue volume by removing some adipocytes or supplementation of stromal vascular fraction or ASCs can increase the ASC/adipocyte ratio in the graft. Clinical results of ASC supplementation remain controversial, but ASC condensation seems to lead to expanding applications of fat grafting into revitalization of stem cell-depleted tissue.

The Authors present three videos of procedures: Video 1 presents chronic wound debridement and fat injections for skin grafting. Video 2 presents fat injection under finger burn wounds. Video 3 presents fat injections under a facial scar

This article presents the authors' 3-year experience with the use of fat grafting, via the Coleman technique, for the adjuvant treatment of burn wounds, venous ulcers, diabetic ulcers, and burn scars. It demonstrates the regenerative effects of fat injected under the scar, and of fat injected under the wound, in the periphery of the wound, and within a bone fracture line or space, and of fat deposited over the wound.

CLINICS IN PLASTIC SURGERY

RELATED INTEREST

Midface and Periocular Rejuvenation
Editor: Anthony P. Sclafani
Facial Plastic Surgery Clinics
May 2015. Volume 23, Issue 2

DOWNLOAD Free App!

Review Articles
THE CLINICS

NOW AVAILABLE FOR YOUR iPhone and iPad

Preface

Fat Grafting: Current Concept, Clinical Application, and Regenerative Potential, Part 1

 CrossMark

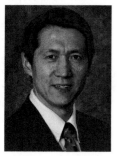 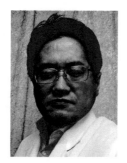 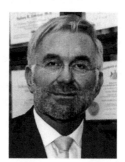

Lee L.Q. Pu, MD, PhD, FACS   Kotaro Yoshimura, MD   Sydney R. Coleman, MD

Editors

Although fat grafting had a "bad reputation" in the past, it has become one of the most commonly performed procedures in both aesthetic and reconstructive plastic surgery. It started as autologous filler for facial rejuvenation, but now it has been used not only for facial rejuvenation but also for breast surgery, body contouring surgery, and other aspects of aesthetic and reconstructive surgery. Until recently, fat grafting has showed its regenerative potential and has been used to treat some of the difficult clinical problems facing plastic surgeons. As we know more about fat grafting, its mechanisms of how fat grafts survive, and their regenerative features, fat grafting as a relatively noninvasive procedure can gradually replace many of the aesthetic and reconstructive procedures in the future. It becomes a major armamentarium for plastic surgeons to rejuvenate aged tissues, to reconstruct a missing part of tissues, to reverse the disease process, and to treat certain pathologic conditions.

Since fat grafting has become a rapidly growing field in plastic surgery with much new advancement for aesthetic and reconstructive surgery, several visionary leaders, including the 3 editors of the issue, have formed a brand new international society, named International Society of Plastic and Regenerative Surgery (ISPRES), in 2011. This young, dynamic international society has gathered many talented plastic surgeons with primary interests and expertise in fat grafting. These 2 issues of *Clinics in Plastic Surgery* are representation of members of this young international organization and their excellent work being presented during the previous world congresses in Rome, Italy, Berlin, Germany, and Miami, USA. Part I of this special issue starts with the history and evolution of fat grafting, followed by the discovery and development of adipose tissue and adipose-derived stem cells. The biology, safety, regulation, and regenerative potential of adipose-derived stem cells are well summarized in this issue. This is followed by the best explanation on how fat grafts survive and remodel and the techniques on how to concentrate stem cells for fat grafting. The good summary on standardizing techniques for fat grafting as well as the update on cryopreservation of fat grafts is also presented in this issue.

Clin Plastic Surg 42 (2015) ix–x
http://dx.doi.org/10.1016/j.cps.2015.02.001
0094-1298/15/$ – see front matter © 2015 Published by Elsevier Inc.

Clinical application of fat grafting for facial rejuvenation, gluteal augmentation, and treatment of burn and burn scars is presented in this issue as well.

We sincerely hope that you will enjoy reading this special issue of *Clinics in Plastic Surgery*. It represents a true team effort from worldwide experts of the ISPRES. We would like to express our heartfelt gratitude to all of the contributors for their expertise, dedication, and responsibility to produce such a world-class monograph of plastic surgery. It is certainly our privilege to work with these respected authors in this exciting field of plastic surgery. We would also like to express our appreciation to the publication team of Elsevier, who has put this remarkable issue together with the highest possible standard.

Lee L.Q. Pu, MD, PhD, FACS
University of California, Davis
Sacramento, CA, USA

Kotaro Yoshimura, MD
University of Tokyo
Tokyo, Japan

Sydney R. Coleman, MD
New York University
New York, NY, USA

University of Pittsburgh
Pittsburgh, PA, USA

E-mail addresses:
lee.pu@ucdmc.ucdavis.edu (L.L.Q. Pu)
kotaro-yoshimura@umin.ac.jp (K. Yoshimura)
sydcoleman@me.com (S.R. Coleman)

History of Fat Grafting
From Ram Fat to Stem Cells

Riccardo F. Mazzola, MD[a],*, Isabella C. Mazzola, MD[b]

KEYWORDS

- History of surgery • History of fat grafting • Fat injection • Regenerative medicine
- Adipose derived stem cells

KEY POINTS

- The first transplantation of adipose tissue from the arm to the orbital region to correct adherent scars from osteomyelitis was performed by Gustav Neuber in 1893.
- The first report of fat injection to the face and breast in the human body to re-establish contour deformities was carried out by Eugene Holländer in 1909.
- In the 1950s, because of its tendency to reabsorb and form oily cysts, fat grafting to the face fell from favor, becoming an almost obsolete procedure.
- With the advent of liposuction, fat injection was rediscovered, but the reabsorption rate was still high.
- In the 1990s, Sydney Coleman systematized the technique for harvesting, purification, and placement of fat, so as to reduce the reabsorption rate.
- In 2001, Zuk and colleagues demonstrated that adipose tissue is the greatest source of adult mesenchymal stem cells, adipose-derived stem cells (ASCs), capable of differentiating into other types of tissues.
- Stromal vascular fraction (SVF), a source of ASCs, endothelial (progenitor) cells, T cells, B cells, mast cells, and adipose tissue macrophages was identified.
- In 2007, Gino Rigotti applied the regenerative properties of ASCs in a human patient. He successfully managed radiation tissue damages, with complete restitutio ad integrum of the affected tissues. This was one of the first examples of regenerative therapies.
- *Fat Injection from Filling to Regeneration*, edited by Sydney Coleman and Riccardo Mazzola, the first textbook that emphasized the regenerative potential of fat in the repair of damaged or missing tissues was published in 2009.

INTRODUCTION

The 19th century is considered the golden age of plastic surgery. A wide array of pedicled skin flaps were described and invented to restore defects, mainly of the face. One of the greatest advances in 19th century surgery was the demonstration that a piece of skin, fully separated from its original site, might survive when transplanted to another part of the body to cover a granulating raw surface. This became possible by the pioneering work of Jacques Reverdin (1842–1929). In 1869, he carried out the first successful epidermic graft on a human patient at Hôpital Necker in Paris, opening a new era in wound management.[1] Skin grafting became soon the preferred solution for the management of chronic wounds.

The Authors have no disclosures.

[a] Department of Clinical Sciences and Community Health, Fondazione Ospedale Maggiore Policlinico IRCCS, Via F. Sforza 35, Milano 20122, Italy; [b] Department of Otolaryngology, Fondazione Ospedale Maggiore Policlinico IRCCS, Via F. Sforza 35, Milano 20122, Italy
* Corresponding author. Via P. Marchiondi 7, Milano 20122, Italy.
E-mail address: riccardo.mazzola@fastwebnet.it

Clin Plastic Surg 42 (2015) 147–153
http://dx.doi.org/10.1016/j.cps.2014.12.002
0094-1298/15/$ – see front matter © 2015 Elsevier Inc. All rights reserved.

THE DISCOVERY OF FAT TRANSPLANTATION: EARLY CLINICAL APPLICATIONS
Fat Transplantation: A New Discovery

Transplantation of tissues, other than skin, was soon attempted. Fat, readily available, was considered the ideal solution to fill in depressions and contour deformities. In 1893, the German surgeon Gustav Neuber (1850–1932) first harvested adipose tissue from the arm and transferred it to the orbital region to correct adherent scar sequelae from osteomyelitis.[2] Shortly afterward, in 1895, another German, Viktor Czerny (1842–1916), transferred a lipoma to the breast to re-establish symmetry, following unilateral partial mastectomy for fibrocystic mastitis.[3]

Fat Grafting

Its indication in the management of the facially disfigured soldiers from World War I
Until introduction of syringes for placing adipose tissue, as it is currently done, fat was always transplanted en-bloc, often with dermis (the so-called dermal fat graft). The healing potentials of fat were empirically noticed by those surgeons who were confronted with the management of the terrible disfigurements caused by World War I. Fat was inserted into the wounds either to promote the healing process or to correct uneven scars from gunshot wounds of soldiers injured in the battlefields. The German maxillofacial surgeon Erich Lexer (1867–1937) first used fat in combination with local flaps and cartilage graft to reconstruct the eye socket so as to accommodate a prosthesis in a facially disfigured soldier (**Fig. 1**). His experience with fat grafting became soon vast. In 1919, he published a 2-volume book "*Die freien Transplantationen*" (Free Transplantations), in which all the different types free grafts available at that time were critically and histologically evaluated.[4] More than 300 pages were devoted to fat grafting, with an incredible range of clinical applications, from the correction of contour deformities for sequelae of facial traumas, to hemifacial microsomia (**Fig. 2**), microgenia, breast asymmetry, post-traumatic hand stiffness and Dupuytren disease to restore the gliding tissue around the tendons. The source of adipose tissue was usually the lateral thigh (**Fig. 3**).

Another surgeon who devoted his skill to the repair of facial disfigurement was Harold Gillies (1882–1960). His book "*Plastic Surgery of the*

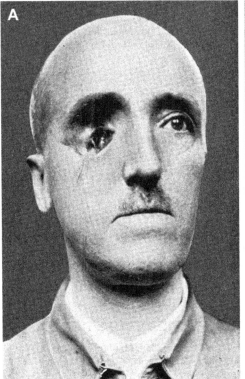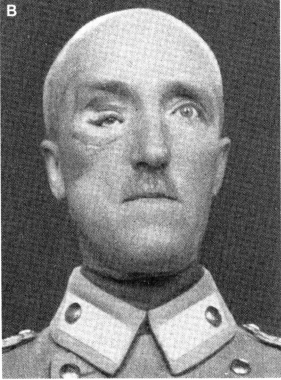

Fig. 1. (*A, B*) Pre- and postoperative view of a soldier injured in World War I, whose eye socket was reconstructed using skin flap, cartilage, and fat graft, so as to accommodate a prosthesis. (*From* Lexer E. Die freien Transplantationen. Stuttgart (Germany): Enke; 1919–1924.)

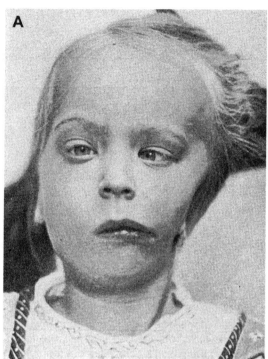
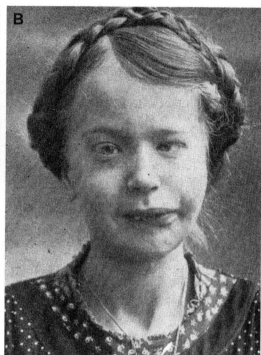

Fig. 2. (*A, B*) Hemifacial microsomia. Assessment at 4 years. (*From* Lexer E. Die freien Transplantationen. Stuttgart (Germany): Enke; 1919–1924.)

Face," published in 1920, showed numerous cases of soldiers from World War I with dramatic facial wounds treated by fat grafting with amazing results (**Fig. 4**).[5]

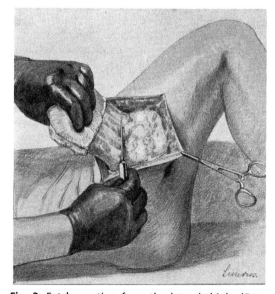

Fig. 3. Fat harvesting from the lateral thigh. (*From* Lexer E. Die freien Transplantationen. Stuttgart (Germany): Enke; 1919–1924.)

The Decline of Fat Transplantation

Initially, surgeons enthusiastically favored the technique of en-bloc fat grafting, alone or in combination with skin flaps, as it often represented the sole way to solve major problems in a simple way. Fat was inserted into the face in case of Romberg disease or into the breast for correct sequelae of mastectomy or to the pharynx to reduce nasal air escape in case of cleft palate surgery.[6] However, in the 1930s, with growing experience, clinicians realized that the encouraging early results worsened over the long term because of an unpredictable reabsorption rate and a tendency to form oily cysts. The pliable fat graft gradually modified, becoming hard and fibrotic.

In the 1950s, Lyndon Peer (1898–1977) investigated the fate of autologous fat transplantation at 1 year and demonstrated that about 50% of fat cells rupture and die after transplantation, and the graft was replaced by fibrous tissue. Cells, which did not rupture, survived and constituted the amount of adipose tissue that remained. He demonstrated that, in autologous fat graft, the new blood circulation establishes at day 4, through anastomosis between blood vessels of the host and those of the graft. If this does not occur, early death of cells may

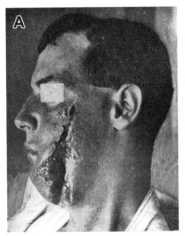
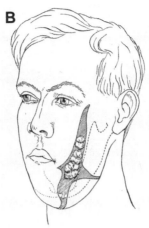
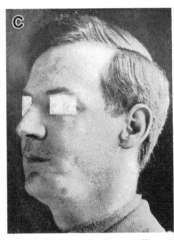

Fig. 4. (*A–C*) Facial wound from World War I. Fat parcels are placed into the wound. Final result. (*From* Gillies HD. Plastic surgery of the face. London: Frowde, Hodder, Stoughton; 1920.)

develop, with oil cyst formation.[7] Because of these considerations, fat grafting to the face fell gradually from favor, turning out to be an almost obsolete procedure.

A REVOLUTIONARY IDEA: INJECTION OF FAT: ITS ORIGIN AND EVOLUTION
Paraffin Injection

At the end of the 19th century, paraffin wax, discovered in 1830 by Baron Carl von Reichenbach (1788–1869), became the first injectable material ever used in modern times. It became popular among beauty doctors to correct depressions, re-establish contour, and modify saddle noses, mainly of syphilitic origin. These unpleasant deformities, charlatans advertised, could be easily improved in beauty salons and drugstores by simple local injections, avoiding any surgical procedure. Disasters appeared soon. Paraffin migrated, causing not only hard swellings, difficult to remove, the so-called paraffinomas, but also pulmonary embolism, infections, and other problems. This recalls the recent story of the injections of liquid silicone, with the devastating adverse effects, the siliconomas, which affected the plastic surgery scenario from the 1960s onwards.

Fat Injection: A Brilliant Idea

To contrast the paraffin complications, in the first decade of the 20th century, the German surgeon Eugene Holländer (1867–1932) had the idea of injecting fat, which he considered a more natural filler. Adipose tissue was obtained from healthy patients. To minimize its reabsorption, the drawback of fat transplantation, Holländer mixed it with a harder type of adipose tissue, harvested from a ram. Then, the specially made cocktail of human and ram, the male fat was moderately heated until it became fluid. Once heated, the mixture was readily available for introduction into the body at blood temperature, so as to improve unpleasant deformities like depressions, facial atrophy (**Fig. 5**) or postmastectomy scars (**Fig. 6**). In his detailed report, Holländer said that patients suffered a painful rash for about 2 to 3 days, but then the postinjection course was uneventful. The technique was published in 1910 and 1912.[8,9]

Fat Injection in the United States

In 1926, in the other side of the Atlantic Ocean, Charles C. Miller (1880–1950) from Chicago, one

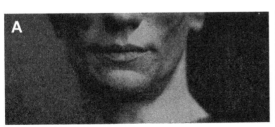
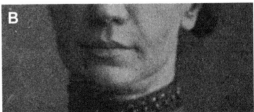

Fig. 5. (*A, B*) Facial atrophy, treated by fat injection. Pre- and post-operative view. (*From* Holländer E. Über einen Fall von fortschreitenden Schwund des Fettgewebes und seinen kosmetischen Ersatz durch Menschenfett. Münch med Wchschr 1910;57:1794–5.)

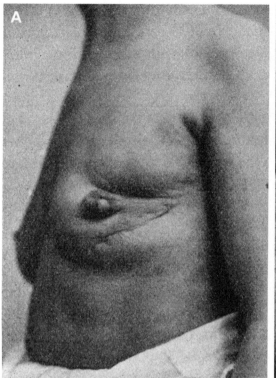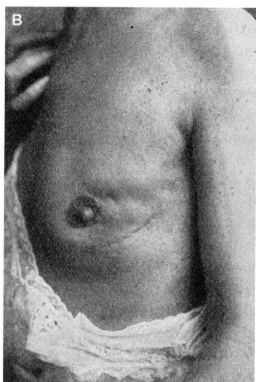

Fig. 6. (*A, B*) Postmastectomy scars treated by fat injection. Pre- and postoperative view. First report of fat injection into the breast. (*From* Holländer E. Über einen Fall von fortschreitenden Schwund des Fettgewebes und seinen kosmetischen Ersatz durch Menschenfett. Münch med Wchschr 1910;57:1794–5.)

of the first US cosmetic surgeons, called either "the father of modern cosmetic surgery" or "an unabashed quack", published *"Cannula Implants"* (**Fig. 7**), a book on fillers to modify featural imperfections.[10] He proposed the use of gutta-percha, celluloid, or rubber sponges grounded in a mill and heated before injecting them to correct depressions, crow's feet, nasolabial grooves, and saddle noses. He asserted that these materials were inert, well tolerated, and particularly effective. Besides these fillers, he harvested a piece of adipose tissue from the abdomen, inserted it into a special screw piston syringe, and injected it subcutaneously to fill in depressions (**Fig. 8**).

However, fat injection never became popular in plastic surgical circles and was seldom employed until the advent of liposuction. On the contrary, for many years paraffin remained the solution of choice for nose and breast augmentation, despite its dramatic consequences.

THE ADVENT OF LIPOSUCTION

In the 1980s, Pierre Fournier[11] and Yves-Gerard Illouz,[12] both from Paris, independently introduced the liposuction, a new procedure for removing fat from the abdomen and thighs of wealthy

overweight Parisian ladies. This technique had an incredible success that spread out all over the world rapidly. On occasion, a too enthusiastic aspiration of fat resulted in unpleasant contour irregularities with depressions and holes. Reintroduction of the lipoaspirate using a syringe was regarded as the solution of choice.[12] But complete or almost complete reabsorption of the reinjected material within a few weeks was reported.

FAT INJECTION BECOMES POPULAR

Despite these unpleasant drawbacks of liposuction, the idea of filling contour depressions concurrent with liposuction using the same adipose tissue just harvested, awakened new interest in autologous fat reinjection.

The Battle Against Reabsorption

At the end of the 1980s, the Argentinean Abel Chajchir published favorable and long-lasting results using fat injection.[13] He considered cautious manipulation of the adipocyte to reduce potential rupture of its fragile cell, rinsing the lipoaspirate in saline to eliminate dead cells and debris and finally grafting fat into close contact with a well

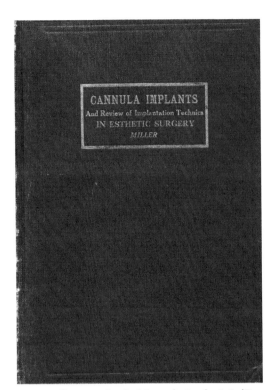

Fig. 7. Miller's textbook *"Cannula Implants."* (*From* Miller CC. Cannula implants and review of implantation technics in esthetic surgery. Chicago: Oak Press; 1926. p. 25–30, 66–71.)

vascularized tissue, crucial steps to minimize reabsorption.

Sydney Coleman and the Systematization of the Technique

In the 1990s, Sydney Coleman systematized the procedure. His recommendations were, harvesting fat using a 3 mm blunt cannula connected to a 10 mL syringe at low negative pressure to decrease adipocyte trauma, purification of the lipoaspirate by means of centrifugation for

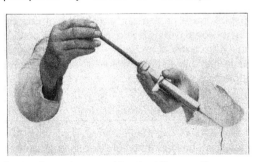

Fig. 8. The syringe used by the US cosmetic surgeon Charles C. Miller for injecting fat. (*From* Miller CC. Cannula implants and review of implantation technics in esthetic surgery. Chicago: Oak Press; 1926. p. 25–30, 66–71.)

separating the oily, aqueous, and adipocyte components, and finally placement in multiple tunnels and in tight contact with a well vascularized surrounding tissue, using a 18G cannula.[14,15] Sydney termed this technique lipostructure.[16]

Fat Injection

The first course in Europe

In 1998, the first course on autologous fat graft was organized in Marseille (France) by Guy Magalon, having Coleman as a guest speaker. This made the diffusion of the technique in Europe easier. At that time, indications for the procedure were mainly correction of contour deformities, postburn scars, Romberg disease, hemifacial microsomia, and chronic soars of the leg.

A few years later, in 2005, Coleman published the first book on fat grafting, in which the procedure of fat grafting was exposed in detail along with numerous clinical applications coming from his experience.[17]

THE ADIPOSE-DERIVED STEM CELLS: A CRUCIAL DISCOVERY

At the beginning of the new millennium, the Pittsburgh team of plastic surgeons and researchers, coordinated by Bill Futrell, made a crucial discovery. They demonstrated that adipose tissue is the greatest source of adult mesenchymal stem cells, the so-called adipose-derived stem cells (ASCs), capable of differentiating into other types of tissue.[18,19] They also identified the stromal vascular fraction (SVF), a source of ASCs, endothelial (progenitor) cells, T cells, B cells, mast cells, and adipose tissue macrophages with repair and regenerative potential, obtained from the lipoaspirates, once the adipose and fluid portion has been removed and processed. This may explain the role of fat grafting in accelerating the healing process and in replacing damaged or missing cells.

Toward Stem Cell Therapy

In 2007, Gino Rigotti and colleagues[20] successfully managed the radiation tissue damages, with complete restitutio ad integrum of the treated tissues, utilizing the regenerative properties of the ASCs. This could be considered the first example of regenerating therapies.

In May 2006, during the 17th Annual Meeting of the European Association of Plastic Surgeons (EURAPS), Riccardo Mazzola, at that time president of the EURAPS, organized the first international panel "Fat Injection, Expanding Opportunities," where the role of fat grafting in the field of regenerative medicine was presented by the faculty with a wide variety of clinical applications. The impact of the panel was significant. The procedure was regarded as one of great clinical value.

That panel evolved the first textbook on this topic, *"Fat Injection from Filling to Regeneration,"* which was published soon afterward and edited by Coleman and Mazzola.[21]

The technique of fat injection spread rapidly, and nowadays meetings, panels and live surgery are continuously organized all over the world. Stem cell therapy, still in its infancy, is fascinating, but it should be approached cautiously. The future is promising. The potential risk of tumorigenicity exists.

SUMMARY

Fat injection empirically started 100 years ago to correct contour deformities mainly on the face and breast. Holländer, who invented the procedure, proposed a cocktail of human and ram fat, to avoid reabsorption.[22,23] Nowadays, fat injection has dramatically evolved, and it ranks among the most popular procedures, for it provides the physician with an incredible range of aesthetic and reconstructive clinical applications with amazing regenerative effects on the surrounding tissues. New research has been made all over the world to demonstrate the role of ASCs, present in the adipose tissue, in the repair of damaged or missing tissues.

REFERENCES

1. Reverdin J. Greffe épidermique. Expérience faite dans le service de M. le Docteur Guyon à l'Hôpital Necker. Bull Soc Imp Chir (Paris) 1869;10:511–5.
2. Neuber G. Über die Wiederanheilung vollständig vom Körper getrennter, die ganze Fettschicht enthaltender Hautstücke. Zbl f Chir 1893;30:16–7.
3. Czerny V. Drei plastische Operationen. III. Plastischer Ersatz der Brustdrüse durch ein Lipom. Arch F Klin Chir 1895;50:544–50.
4. Lexer E. Die freien Transplantationen. Stuttgart (Germany): Enke; 1919–1924.
5. Gillies HD. Plastic surgery of the face. London: Frowde, Hodder, Stoughton; 1920.
6. Gaza von W. Über freie Fettgewebstransplantation in den retropharyngealen Raum bei Gaumenspalte. Arch F Klin Chir 1926;142:590–9.
7. Peer LA. Transplantation of tissues. Baltimore (MD): Williams & Wilkins; 1955.
8. Holländer E. Über einen Fall von fortschreitenden Schwund des Fettgewebes und seinen kosmetischen Ersatz durch Menschenfett. Münch Med Wochenschr 1910;57:1794–5.
9. Holländer E. Die kosmetische Chirurgie. In: Joseph M, editor. Handbuch der Kosmetik. Leipzig (Germany): von Veit; 1912. p. 689–90, 708.
10. Miller CC. Cannula implants and review of implantation technics in esthetic surgery. Chicago: Oak Press; 1926. p. 25–30, 66–71.
11. Fournier PF. Microlipoextraction et microlipoinjection. Rev Cir Esthét Langue 1985;10:36–40.
12. Illouz YG. The fat cell "graft": a new technique to fill depressions. Plast Reconstr Surg 1986;78:122–3.
13. Chajchir A, Benzaquen I. Fat-grafting injection for soft-tissue augmentation. Plast Reconstr Surg 1989;84:921–34.
14. Coleman SR. The technique of periorbital lipoinfiltration. Oper Techn Plast Surg 1994;1:120–6.
15. Coleman SR. Long-term survival of fat transplants: controlled demonstrations. Aesthetic Plast Surg 1995;19:421–5.
16. Coleman SR. Facial recontouring with lipostructure. Clin Plast Surg 1997;24:347–67.
17. Coleman SR. Structural fat grafting. St Louis (MO): Quality Medical Publishing; 2005.
18. Zuk PA, Zhu M, Mizuno H, et al. Multilineage cells from human adipose tissue: implications for cell-based therapies. Tissue Eng 2001;7:211–28.
19. Zuk PA, Zhu M, Ashjian P, et al. Human adipose tissue is a source of multipotent stem cells. Mol Biol Cell 2002;13:4279–95.
20. Rigotti G, Marchi A, Galié M, et al. Clinical treatment of radiotherapy tissue damage by lipoaspirate transplant: a healing process mediated by adipose-derived adult stem cells. Plast Reconstr Surg 2007;119:1409–22.
21. Coleman SR, Mazzola RF. Fat injection from filling to regeneration. St Louis (MO): Quality Medical Publishing; 2009.
22. Mazzola RF. The evolution of fat grafting: from soft tissue augmentation to regenerative medicine. In: Coleman SR, Mazzola RF, editors. Fat injection from filling to regeneration. St Louis (MO): Quality Medical Publishing; 2009. p. XIX–XXXVIII.
23. Mazzola RF, Mazzola IC. The fascinating history of fat grafting. J Craniofac Surg 2013;24:1069–71.

Adipose Tissue and Stem/Progenitor Cells
Discovery and Development

Sahil K. Kapur, MD[a], Severiano Dos-Anjos Vilaboa, PhD[b],
Ramon Llull, MD, PhD[b], Adam J. Katz, MD[c],*

KEYWORDS

- Adipose • Adipose stem cells • Stromal vascular fraction • Cell therapy • Regeneration

KEY POINTS

- Adipose tissue is a valuable, exploitable, appealing source of regenerative cells.
- Adipose tissue can be used for a variety of clinical challenges.
- Adipose tissue has entered clinical testing throughout the world and has been shown to be safe and feasible in a variety of models.
- Commercial infrastructure/scalability of cell manufacturing is nearing the tipping point.
- Adipose-derived therapies can be developed for clinical use in a variety of ways.
- Adipose-derived therapies will be developed in waves of complexity.
- Current approaches seem to be influenced by regulatory considerations as much as by scientific considerations.

INTRODUCTION

Previously perceived as worthless and unwanted, adipose tissue has emerged over the last 15 years as a premiere source of cells for evolving tissue engineering and regenerative therapies. It was once thought to function merely as padding for internal organs, nerves, and vessels, but now adipose tissue is known to be a complex, dynamic, bioactive organ that is involved in a diverse array of physiologic and disease processes. In the 1960s, Rodbell[1,2] described the dissociation and separation of adipose tissue into a single cell suspension, enabling and ushering in a new era of study of its different cellular components. This subsequently manifested as an expanded understanding of the adipocyte precursor cell (ie, the preadipocyte) and its differentiation program.[3–5] In the 1980s and 1990s, the cellular constituents of adipose tissue became a central topic of study

within the context of obesity, and eventually for the study and understanding of fat grafting.[6–8] Ultimately, the preadipocyte became a focal point for the emerging field of tissue engineering.[9–13]

As the cellular diversity of adipose tissue became more appreciated, interest in its use as a cell source increased. As early as 1986, Jarrell and colleagues[14] published on the isolation and use of adipose-derived microvascular endothelial cells for lining synthetic vascular grafts.[15] By the turn of the century, the idea that adipose tissue contained progenitor/stem cells with the ability to differentiate into lineages other than adipocytes emerged. In 2000, Halvorsen and colleagues[16] described the osteogenic differentiation of adipose-derived stromal cells, and in 2001 Zuk and colleagues[17] published findings showing that adipose tissue was a novel source of mesenchymal stem cells (MSCs) with multilineage differentiation potential. There is now a large body of

[a] Division of Plastic and Reconstructive Surgery, University of Wisconsin, Madison, Madison, WI, USA; [b] Stem Center, Cami dels Reis 308, Palma de Mallorca 07010, Spain; [c] Department of Surgery, University of Florida College of Medicine, 1600 SW Archer Road, Gainesville, FL 32610, USA
* Corresponding author.
E-mail address: adam.katz@surgery.ufl.edu

Clin Plastic Surg 42 (2015) 155–167
http://dx.doi.org/10.1016/j.cps.2014.12.010
0094-1298/15/$ – see front matter © 2015 Elsevier Inc. All rights reserved.

plasticsurgery.theclinics.com

literature to suggest that a wide variety of tissues may contain an MSC fraction. To this end, Crisan and colleagues,[18] as well as several other independent groups, have proposed a unifying theory that MSCs from various organs/tissues are located in the perivascular space/niche.[19,20] The notion that pericytes (also called mural cells, or Rouget cells) have multilineage potential is not new, and dates back at least to the early 1980s.[21–25] Furthermore, the unique microvascular composition of adipose tissue has been appreciated for at least a quarter of a century, if not longer.[26–28]

The growing global interest in the use of adipose tissue as a source of cells, matrix, and factors for regenerative and tissue engineering purposes is readily manifest in a simple PubMed literature search. As shown in **Fig. 1**, the number of peer-reviewed publications involving the key words "adipose" and "stem cells" has increased greatly since 2001. A similar pattern of growth is evident in a search of the National Institutes of Health clinical trial site, www.clinicaltrials.gov, with similar terms. Coincident with these basic science and translational research advancements, a novel field or discipline emerged related to the therapeutic application of adipose-derived components (eg, cells, matrix, soluble factors). In addition, the growth and maturation of this field has created a need for an enabling clinical infrastructure that is now evident in the form of an expanding market opportunity for new and existing commercial entities. One of the major driving factors behind this commercial interest is the now full realization by the broader community of stakeholders that adipose tissue is unrivaled in its abundance, safety, appeal, and ease in terms of its harvest.

CELL IDENTITY AND TERMINOLOGY

The stromal vascular fraction (SVF) is defined as a heterogeneous population of freshly isolated cells from adipose tissue after enzymatic dissociation (**Figs. 2** and **3**). This cell population is composed of many different stromal cell types, such as

Cell Isolation from Adipose Tissue

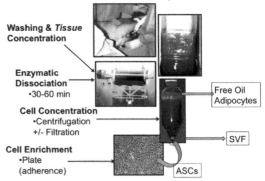

Fig. 2. The basic steps of cell isolation from liposuction harvested adipose tissue, and the resulting cell fractions. ASCs, adipose stromal/stem cells.

vascular progenitors, fibroblasts, pericytes, or mesenchymal stromal cells, but excluding mature adipocytes.[29] Within the SVF, the stromal cells of interest comprise approximately 20% of the cell fraction and have the markers CD45-, CD235a-, CD31-, CD34+; and the surface antigens CD13, CD73, CD90, CD105. In contrast, adipose stromal/stem cells (ASCs) are plastic adherent culture-expanded cells derived from SVF that possess the capability of differentiation into different mesenchymal lineages and positive expression for several immunophenotypic markers (CD90, CD105, CD73, CD44, and so forth) and are negative for CD45 and CD31 (**Fig. 3, Table 1**).[29] They share these markers with other MSCs but can be differentiated from bone marrow mesenchymal stem cells (BM-MSC) based on CD36 positivity and CD 106 negativity. Furthermore, studies have suggested that ASCs have a greater propensity of differentiating into muscle tissue compared with MSCs. In contrast, MSCs have been observed to more readily differentiate into chondrogenic and osteogenic lineages.[29,30]

In short, subcutaneous human adipose tissue is an accessible and abundant cell source for regenerative medicine applications. Researchers and biotech companies have explored different methods and point-of-care devices to isolate regenerative cells from human adipose lipoaspirates obtained from liposuction procedures. The body of literature has provided evidence about safety and efficacy of fresh SVF cells and cultured ASCs using in vivo animal models, as well as in different clinical studies and case reports.[31–35]

Differentiation Potential

In vitro studies using human and rodent ASCs have effectively shown the trilineage differentiation

Publications

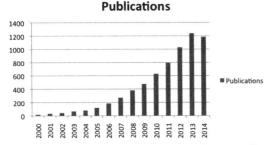

Fig. 1. PubMed search for "adipose" and "stem cell." Number of publications is listed on the Y axis. Note: 2014 citations do not reflect a full year.

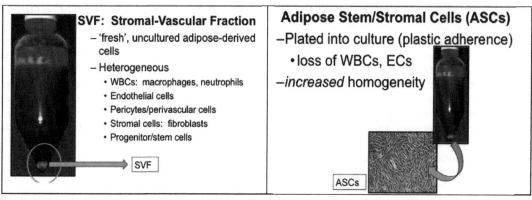

Fig. 3. SVF versus ASCs. SVF cells are a primary, mixed, uncultured cell population. ASCs have been plated into culture, and become purified based on selection by adherence. EC, endothelial cells; WBC, white blood cell.

Table 1
Literature summary of cell surface markers for ASCs

Authors, Reference, Year	Positive Expression	Negative Expression
Gronthos et al,[110] 2001	CD9, CD10, CD13, CD29, CD34, CD44 CD49d, CD49e, CD54, CD55, CD59 CD105, CD146, CD166, HLA-ABC	CD11a, CD11b, CD11c, CD31, CD45 CD50, CD56, CD62e, HLA-DR
Zuk et al,[17] 2001	CD13, CD29, CD44, CD49d, CD71	CD14, CD16, CD31, CD34, CD45
Zuk et al,[111] 2002	CD90, CD105, STRO-1, SH3	CD56, CD62e, CD104, CD106, SMA
Katz et al,[112] 2005	CD29, CD49b, CD49d, CD49e, CD51 CD61, CD90, CD138, CDl40a	CD11a, CD11b, CD11c, CD18, CD41a CD49f, CD62L, CD62P, CD106 CD117, CD133, HLA-DR, ABC
Mitchell et al,[113] 2006	CD13, CD29, CD34, CD44, CD49a CD63, CD73, CD90, CD146, CD166	CD31, CD144
Yoshimura et al,[114] 2006	CD34, CD90	CD31, CD45, CD105, CD146
Oedayrajsingh-Varma et al,[115] 2007	CD34, CD54, CD90, CD105, CD117 HLA-ABC, HLA-DR	CD31, CD45, CD106, CD146, CD166
Zannettino et al,[20] 2008	CD44, CD90, CD105, CD106, CD146 CD166, STRO-1, 3G5	CD14, CD31, CD45
Traktuev et al,[116] 2008	CD10, CD13, CD34, CD90, CDl40a CD140b, SMA	CD31, CD45, CD144
Zimmerlin et al,[117] 2010	CD34, CD90	CD31, CD146, SMA
Lin et al,[118] 2008	CD34	CD31, CDl40b, SMA
Proposed phenotype of ASCs (common between 2 or more studies)	CD13, CD29, CD34, CD44, CD49d CD54, CD90, CD140a, HLA-ABC	CD11a, CD11b, CD11c, CD14, CD31 CD45, CD106, CD144
Controversial markers in ASCs	CD105, CDl40b, CD146, CD166, SMA HLA-DR	—
Stromal cell markers	CD29, CD44, CD73, CD90, CD166	—
Hematopoietic markers	CD31, CD34, CD45, ABCG2	—
Pericyte markers	CD146, Stro-1, 3G5	—

Markers in common between studies shown in bold.

Abbreviations: 3G5, pericyte marker; ABCG2, multidrug transporter protein G2; HLA, human leukocyte antigen; SMA, smooth muscle actin.

From Zuk P. Adipose-derived stem cells in tissue regeneration: a review. Stem Cells 2013;2013:35. [Hindawi Publishing Corporation. Article ID: 713959].

potential of these cells. ASCs induced with dexamethasone undergo osteogenic differentiation leading to production of various growth factors similar to mature cells of this phenotype.[36] Osteogenic differentiation is also seen in ASCs grown in two-dimensional and three-dimensional (3D) tissue engineered constructs using materials such as collagen, poly lactic-co-glycolic acid (PLGA), carbon nanotubes, silk sponges, or self-assembling spheroids (**Fig. 4**).[37–38] Furthermore, successful osteogenic differentiation is also seen in ASCs isolated from 24-hour-old cadaveric tissue.[39] In vivo osteogenic differentiation of ASCs has been successfully shown in calvarial, maxillo-mandibular, and long bone defects. Preinduction of ASCs using dexamethasone/VD3 (1,25-dihydroxyvitamin D3) greatly improve the osteogenic capabilities of these cells compared with uninduced ASCs.[40] The use of ASCs treated with bone morphogenetic protein 2 (BMP2) in improving bone production has shown promising results; however, there continues to be controversy about whether similar effects can be achieved by using BMP alone.[41–43]

Chondrogenic differentiation is seen in ASCs grown in induction media containing members of the transforming growth factor beta family and in ASCs seeded on multiple tissue engineering constructs.[44] In vivo chondrogenic differentiation using preinduced ASCs or ASCs transfected with

TGF beta have shown production of cartilage in various in vivo models.[45] Studies showing the successful production of articular cartilage and integration with recipient cartilage in animal models show promising clinical potential.[43,46]

ASC differentiation into mature fat has been shown in in vivo models in which mature adipose tissue is generated from transplantation of green fluorescent protein (GFP)-labeled ASCs.[47] Multiple studies also advocate the supplementation of fat grafts with ASCs to help increase take and prolong the longevity and volume retention of the grafted tissue.[48]

Eom and colleagues[49] showed differentiation of ASCs into skeletal muscle cells using 5-azacytidine and basic fibroblast growth factor (bFGF) induction agents. Differentiation of ASCs into myotubes has been seen when cells are grown in conjunction with myoblasts and on mechanically patterned surfaces.[50] Successful differentiation of ASCs into smooth muscle cells and mature cardiac myocytes has been shown by the expression of mature phenotype-specific and lineage-specific markers in these cells.[51,52]

In vivo differentiation in skeletal muscle tissue has been shown in studies using a subpopulation of ASCs that had been produced by rapid adherence to tissue culture polystyrene. Preinduced ASCs preferentially homed to injured muscle tissue. The cells expressed the expected muscle

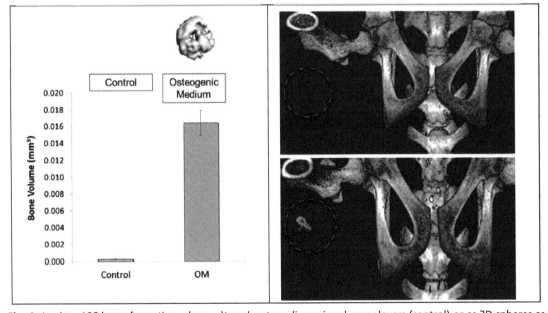

Fig. 4. In vitro ASC bone formation when cultured as two-dimensional monolayers (control) or as 3D spheres as measured by micro–computed tomography (*left*). Similar results are found 2 weeks after implantation in vivo with monolayer cultured cells (*top right*), and 3D spheroid implants shown bottom right. (*From* Shen FH, Werner BC, Liang H, et al. Implications of adipose-derived stromal cells in a 3D culture system for osteogenic differentiation: an in vitro and in vivo investigation. Spine J 2013;13(1):32–43; with permission.)

differentiation markers, including MyoD, myogenin, myosin, and dystrophin, along with good engraftment into target muscle tissue.[53,54] Similar regenerative effects of ASCs have been seen with respect to smooth muscle cell and cardiomyocyte differentiation. Preinduced ASCs were shown to differentiate into urinary bladder smooth muscle cells and, when injected in combination with nerve growth factor, ASCs resulted in improved bladder capacity and reduced stress urinary incontinence in rats.[55] Decreased apoptosis and increased angiogenesis were promoted in a diabetic bladder model injected with ASCs.[56] ASCs increased left ventricular ejection fraction and improved vascularization of infarcted cardiac tissue by directly differentiating into cardiac myocytes and via expression of proangiogenic growth factors and cytokines (vascular endothelial growth factor [VEGF], bFGF, TGFb).[43,57,58]

Ectodermal differentiation of ASCs has been shown by the creation of neurospheres and cells expressing neuronal markers (neuron-specific enolase [NSE], NeuN, nestin, microtubule-associated protein 2 [MAP2], tau, beta-tubulin III, Nkx2.2, Pax6, Olig2) and neuronlike phenotypes (delayed rectifier K currents and tetrodotoxin (TTX) sensitive sodium currents).[59,60] In vivo studies have shown ASC-mediated regeneration in both central and peripheral nervous system models. ASCs reduced infarct size when injected into areas of ischemic stroke in a rodent stroke model. Improvement in extremity function and neural conduction velocities were also seen with ASC transplantation into areas of spinal contusion.[61,62] In a peripheral nerve injury model, acellular conduits loaded with ASCs led to neural regeneration comparable with the gold standard of regeneration via autografts.[63] ASCs have also been successfully induced down epidermal lineage pathways to generate epithelial-like cells and dermal stroma capable of supporting proliferation and differentiation of keratinocyte cultures.[64,65]

IMMUNOMODULATION

Although differentiation-specific uses have great potential and use in tissue regeneration, ASCs also exert significant immunomodulatory effects. They have been shown to increase secretion of interleukin (IL)-6, IL-10, IL-4, and GCSF, and to stimulate proliferation of regulatory and helper T-cell phenotypes. ASC-mediated immunosuppression has led to beneficial antiinflammatory effects in hemorrhagic stroke and reactive airway disease animal models.[66,67] Early results from phase III clinical trials using ASCs in the treatment of inflammatory bowel disease have shown increased healing of

fistulas without any significant side effects.[68] ASC treatments have led to improved neurologic function in patients with multiple sclerosis as well as improvements in other autoimmune disorder–related conditions such as hearing loss and rheumatoid arthritis.[69,70] These successes have prompted investigation into the role ASCs could play in the prolongation of transplant-related immunosuppressive therapy and in the suppression of graft-versus-host disease.[43,71]

SECRETOME

ASCs modify their environment via direct differentiation into target tissue cells as well as via secretion of cytokines and growth factors that exert paracrine effects. Ischemic limb model experiments comparing the effects of transplanted ASC cells with conditioned ASC media show that ASC media (containing high levels of granulocyte colony stimulating factor (GCSF), TGFB, VEGF, hepatocyte growth factor [HGF], and fibroblast growth factor [FGF]) exert similar, albeit less intense, angiogenic effects on the ischemic tissue.[72] Similar paracrine effects of ASC-mediated proangiogenic factors have been shown in acute myocardial injury models.[73] Immunoregulatory effects of ASC-conditioned media have been shown by the suppression of peripheral blood mononuclear cells through modulation of interferon gamma, HGF, prostaglandin E2 (PGE2), TGFB-1, indoleamine 2,3-dioxygenase (IDO), and IL-10.[74] These effects are gaining importance in developing novel treatment modalities for Crohn disease, multiple sclerosis, and graft-versus-host disease.[62,69,75–77] Conditioned media generated under proinflammatory stimuli have also shown improved wound healing rates in rodent wound healing models via the attraction of monocytes to sites of inflammation and tissue damage. Tissue regeneration via extracellular matrix (ECM) remodelling, keratinocyte migration, and increase in capillary density has been seen with the application of ASC-secreted cytokines (CTFG, SERPINE1, PAI, HGF, and FGF-1).[78–81] In addition to the mechanisms summarized earlier, ASCs may also exert biological effects via direct cell-cell contacts. For example, ASCs can affect microvascular density and stability by acting as pericytes. Mendel and colleagues showed this elegantly in the context of 2 different murine models of retinopathy (**Fig. 5**).

Scaffold-free spheroid preparation of ASCs generates media that exert more potent effects on wound healing rates than media generated by ASCs grown in monolayers. Media from 3D ASC preparations generate large amounts of ECM-related factors in addition to growth

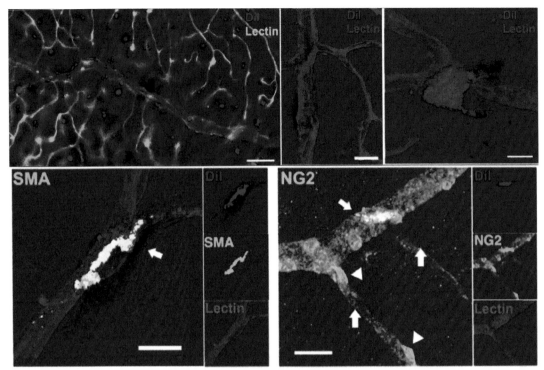

Fig. 5. (*Top*) DiI (1,1′-dioctadecyl-3,3,3′,3′-tetramethylindocarbocyanine perchlorate; a fluorescent membrane stain)-labeled (*red*) human ASCs (hASCs) injected intravitreally at postnatal day 12 (P12) following oxygen-induced retinopathy (OIR) home from the vitreous to murine retinal microvasculature (*green*) as seen following harvest at P22. DiI-labeled hASCs (*red*) wrap around isolectin-labeled retinal microvessels (*blue*) abluminally and target vascular junctions, both properties of terminally differentiated pericytes. (*Bottom*) DiI-labeled hASCs injected intravitreally into NOD (nonobese diabetic [mouse strain]) SCID (severe combined immunodeficient [mouse strain]) mice at P12, after OIR hyperoxia, maintain intimate association with the retinal microvasculature 6 to 8 weeks later and show persistent smooth muscle actin (SMA), NG2 (neural/glical antigen 2, often used as a marker of pericyte cells; *white arrows*), with SMA extending into the cellular extension wrapping around the capillary. (*Modified from* Mendel TA, Clabough EB, Kao DS, et al. Pericytes derived from adipose-derived stem cells protect against retinal vasculopathy. PLoS One 2013;8(5):e65691.)

factors that promote tissue regeneration. The synergistic effects of both ECM proteins and these growth factors are considered to be one of the possible reasons for the more potent benefits observed.[82–84]

In addition to relying on the innate ability of ASCs to differentiate or secrete factors in their target environment, their behavior can be engineered to secrete large amounts of specific growth factors, allowing them to behave like biopumps. The osteogenic properties of ASCs can be augmented by transducing these cells to increase production of BMP2, BMP4, BMP6, and TGF B2.[85] Similarly, ASCs can be transduced to secrete large amounts of VEGF and brain-derived neurotrophic factor to help improve their angiogenic properties. The tumor trophic properties of these cells have been used to transmit oncolytic factors and treat gliomas.[86] ASC cells can be converted into natural killer–like cells via the

transduction of natural killer cell transcription factors in hematopoietically induced ASCs. These cells have successfully shown tumor killing properties and slowed progression of breast cancer and prostate cancer cells in a nude murine model.[87] ASCs from both fresh and cyropreserved sources have been modified into induced pluripotent stem cells via expression of known stemness genes (Oct4, Sox2, Klf4, and c-myc).[88,89] These cells form embryoid bodies in vitro that express germ cell markers including desmin, vimentin, GFAP, alpha fetoprotein, and Sox17. They assume properties of embryonic stem cells and are capable of multilineage differentiation. Dedifferentiation of mature adipocytes has been shown to produce a more potent source of ASCs. These cells retain most of the known properties of ASCs, such as their capability of multilineage differentiation, and also express stemness genes (oct4, sox2 c-myc, and Nanog).[43,90]

DEVELOPMENT OF CELL-BASED THERAPIES

For those cell therapies using adipose tissue as a cell source there is debate about the potency and clinical application of the different cell populations that can be derived (ie, SVF cells vs ASCs). Among the different factors affecting decision making, the most important are the regulatory requirements needed, the availability of approved facilities, cell dose requirements, associated costs, and processing time. There has been much more research performed in the past addressing the characterization, biology, and therapeutic potential of ASCs than of SVF cells.[91–94]

However, there has recently been an emerging focus on the biology and clinical translation of SVF cells. The use of autologous freshly isolated SVF cells at the point of care in real time during a same surgical procedure has important advantages with respect to the use of culture-expanded cells: less chance for contamination, more rapid processing and clinical application, and fewer associated costs. Some disadvantages that have previously been reported are insufficient cell dose if high cell numbers are needed, and lack of efficacy. Nevertheless, there are few studies in the literature directly comparing the efficacy/potency of SVF cells versus ASCs using different experimental models. Furthermore, it is also important to emphasize that many published reports inaccurately use the terms ASCs or adipose stem cells to refer to SVF.

Several studies show improved results with freshly obtained stromal cells compared with cultured cells. For example, Semon and colleagues[95] reported that an intraperitoneal dose of 1 million SVF cells was more effective than ASCs in inhibiting experimental autoimmune encephalomyelitis progression. Autologous SVF cells also had a more evident positive effect (improvement of range of motion and pain for all patients) than allogeneic ASCs in a model of hip dysplasia in dogs.[96] However, the investigators stated that further studies are necessary (because of small sample size) to assess a clear advantage of SVF cells in treating joint diseases. In another study, Jurgens and colleagues[97] showed best performance of freshly isolated SVF cells compared with cultured ASCs in promoting cartilage and subchondral bone regeneration in a goat model. All of these studies have shown safety and feasibility of point-of-care SVF cell therapies with no adverse effects related to the treatments reported.

In summary, it remains to be determined whether putative functional differences between SVF cells and ASCs have relevance for specific clinical applications. Additional preclinical data and clinical trials comparing both cell types may help to clarify these questions.

CURRENT GAPS AND CONTROVERSIES: TUMORIGENESIS

Considerable controversy exists in the literature with regard to the behavior of ASCs and tumors. ASCs, and more generally MSCs, have been found to show tumor tropism leading to engraftment of cells in the tumor mass, increase in size of the tumor mass, and development of fibrovascular stroma more permissive for tumor growth and metastasis.[98]

Meulberg and colleagues[99] studied the effects of tissue-resident ASCs and injected ASCs in a syngeneic mouse model. They showed tumor tropism and tumor-promoting effects of both ASC populations. Based on their deductions, the ASCs showed their tumorigenic effects via the SDF-1/CXCL-4 receptor interactions. Furthermore ASCs led to increased vascular density around the tumors and assimilated in tumor blood vessels. Repeated experiments with human breast cancer cells and human ASCs showed similar results. ASCs coinjected with lung tumor and glioma cells in a nude mouse model also showed increase in tumor size and cell viability.[100]

Tumor-promoting effects of ASCs were also shown in a study of human breast cancer cells characterized from malignant pleural effusions. Coculturing these tumor cells with ASCs led to a 5.1-fold increased in tumor proliferation rate. ASCs also had a more potent tumorigenic effect on active malignant cells compared with cells in a resting state.[101]

Another group analyzed the tumor tropism of SVF cells in a mouse Lewis lung carcinoma model and mice transplanted with breast adenocarcinoma, prostate adenocarcinoma, and Kaposi sarcoma xenografts. SVF cells homed to tumors, engrafted within tumors, and speeded up tumor growth. They were also able to distinguish 2 major components of SVF: ASCs and adipose-derived endothelial cells. Both of these populations showed tumor tropism and engrafted in separate niches within the tumor. SVF cells injected both intravenously and subcutaneously migrated to tumors. Furthermore, the group found that even white adipose implants led to tumor growth via the recruitment of stromal cells from the grafts. Paracrine effects of SPARC (secreted protein acidic and rich in cysteine) and its interaction with cell surface marker CD29 was implicated in the homing mechanism.[102]

Conditioned media from adipose-derived stem cells when cocultured with endometrial cancer cells led to increased proliferation of these cancer cells.

These cancer cells produced 10% more VEGF when cultured in ASC-conditioned media taken from patients with cancer compared with ASC-conditioned media from cancer-free controls.[103] Another recent study showed that coculture of ASC and inflammatory breast cancer cells (T47D) increased production of tumorigenic cytokines, specifically IL-6, IL-10, IL-2, GCSF, and IL-1alpha. Imaging of the coculture using electromicrography revealed that the tumor cells had attained a characteristic tumorsphere phenotype and had developed filopodia-mediated connections with surrounding ASCs. Furthermore, immunofluorescence studies showed exosomal vesicular transfer between ASCs and tumor cells. The coculture environment promoted the development of malignant tumor marker and regulatory genes signifying epithelial to mesenchymal transition and a more invasive cancer phenotype. These genes included EpCam, Erb2, Lef1, FGFR1, and SNCG.[104]

Although the studies discussed earlier implicate ASCs in tumor progression, multiple studies describe an opposite, antitumor effect of adipose-derived cells. Zhu and colleagues[105] clearly showed the inhibitory effects on human ASCs on hematopoietic tumor cells and breast cancer cells. In vitro coculture studies showed a reduction in cell proliferation activity of up to 80% in hematopoietic cells and up to 60% in breast cancer cells. These tumor suppressive effects were also seen when tumor cells and ASCs were coimplanted in a humoral microenvironment (created using implanted CellMax® artificial capillary modules) in nude mice. Furthermore, cells taken from patients with chronic myelogenous leukemia showed a reduction in cell proliferation rate when cocultured with ASCs. The antitumor effects were noted to be caused by paracrine secretion of DKK-1 by the ASCs. DKK-1 is a potent inhibitor of the beta-catenin pathway, and has also been implicated in MSC-related tumor suppression in other studies.[106]

Sun and colleagues[107] showed beneficial use of human ASCs in a murine breast cancer model. They effectively showed that ASCs injected into a murine model about 22 days following the development of breast cancer (via injection of breast cancer cells into the inguinal fat pad) caused a significant reduction in tumor size. They also showed that ASC injection led to a reduction in lung cancer metastases. They proposed that ASCs promoted apoptosis via poly ADP ribose polymerase (PARP) cleavage and production of caspase-3 leading to tumor cell death.

Given the contradictory findings in tumor behavior in response to ASCs, and the antitumor effects seen in humoral malignancies, Cousin and colleagues[108] further explored ASC effects on

solid tumors by studying the behavior of pancreatic ductal adenocarcinoma cells in the presence of ASCs. In vitro cocultures of tumor cells with ASCs showed a 40% decrease in proliferation rate. Similar effects were seen when ASCs were injected into pancreatic ductal carcinoma masses in an in vivo murine model. The group also observed that ASC-conditioned media showed antitumor effects. Similar antitumor effects were not seen by BM-MSC–conditioned media. Further analysis suggested that ASCs exerted their effects by downregulating CDK4, leading to G1-phase arrest followed by cell necrosis without apoptosis.

Despite numerous experimental studies, there continues to be significant controversy regarding the role of ASCs in tumorigenesis. This controversy is to be expected given the heterogeneity of mechanisms and scenarios that lead to tumor development and progression compounded with the heterogeneous effects that ASCs exert on their environment. Furthermore, adipose-derived cells could simultaneously promote and inhibit tumor growth by inhibiting cellular processes leading to tumor progression and concurrently creating an immunosuppressive environment that is tumor protective. Although there continues to be confusion regarding the role of adipose-derived stem cells and SVF in the promotion or inhibition of tumors, findings from the RESTORE-2 clinical trial show no cancer recurrences (in a 12-month period) in any of the subjects receiving fat grafts augmented by SVF and ASCs for reconstruction following breast conservation therapy.[109]

Obstacles to Development: Regulatory and Commercialization Risk

Cell-based regenerative medicine, like any other medical treatment, must fulfill minimal requirements to be used in humans, the most important being patient safety, followed by clinical efficacy.

The clinical use of cells (freshly isolated or not) is being regulated by the different regulatory agencies around the world, and the regulatory framework depends on the country. The European Medicines Agency (EMA) in Europe, The Food and Drug Administration (FDA) in the United States, and other regional authorities have developed different guidelines and laws to regulate this emerging field, in order to protect patient safety. In general, the cellular products to be used in patients can be classified into those that are autologous, minimally manipulated, and reinjected during the same surgical act (ie, freshly isolated SVF cells), or those that are substantially manipulated (ie, cultured-expanded ASCs autologous or allogeneic). Another important point being considered is the concept that cells should be used in a manner consistent with their normal essential function.

One frustrating theme for translational researchers is that the regulatory framework is being continuously revised and updated to be compliant with new available clinical data and scientific findings. As an example, the EMA Committee for Advanced Therapies (CAT) has recently released a reflection paper for public consultation with some proposed changes to current regulation of cell therapies in Europe. Specifically, the committee has recently released a reflection paper on the classification of advanced-therapy medicinal products (ATMPs) to reflect the current thinking of the committee on how ATMPs should be classified, including a change to the definition of substantial manipulation. Until now, in Europe the use of collagenase as a way to isolate cells during the same surgical act and for the same individual (autologous) was classified as a cell separation method, and hence included in the list of nonsubstantial manipulations of regulation EC 1394/2007. In this reflection paper the EMA-CAT is studying the possibility of classifying enzymatic digestion as a substantial manipulation. Because this change would reflect a position more similar to current FDA policy in the United States, this may reflect growing momentum of efforts by global regulatory bodies to establish an international harmonization of policies governing cell therapies.

SUMMARY

The clinical application of ASCs and SVF cells is just beginning to gain momentum. Important progress has been made in the last several years. It is clear that adipose-derived cells may mediate therapeutic effects through a multitude of mechanisms, but paracrine-mediated signaling of angiogenesis, inflammation, cell homing, cell survival, and similar processes have emerged as primary mechanisms of action. As the scientific understanding of these cells increases, the regulatory framework that governs their clinical use also matures. In addition, although specific regulatory rules currently depend on a given country, there seems to be a trend (or at least an effort) toward the unification of policies across the globe. In addition, there are now multiple companies ushering novel, enabling cell isolation devices through the regulatory process. The maturation of science, regulatory policy and commercial infrastructure along with scalability are leading to an important inflection point in the development and translation of this promising field.

REFERENCES

1. Rodbell M. Localization of lipoprotein lipase in fat cells of rat adipose tissue. J Biol Chem 1964;239: 753–5.
2. Rodbell M. Metabolism of isolated fat cells. I. Effects of hormones on glucose metabolism and lipolysis. J Biol Chem 1964;239:375–80.
3. Loffler G, Hauner H. Adipose tissue development: the role of precursor cells and adipogenic factors. Part II: the regulation of the adipogenic conversion by hormones and serum factors. Klin Wochenschr 1987;65(17):812–7.
4. Teichert-Kuliszewska K, Hamilton BS, Deitel M, et al. Augmented production of heparin-binding mitogenic proteins by preadipocytes from massively obese persons. J Clin Invest 1992; 90(4):1226–31.
5. Petruschke T, Hauner H. Tumor necrosis factor-alpha prevents the differentiation of human adipocyte precursor cells and causes delipidation of newly developed fat cells. J Clin Endocrinol Metab 1993;76(3):742–7.
6. Hauner H, Entenmann G. Regional variation of adipose differentiation in cultured stromal-vascular cells from the abdominal and femoral adipose tissue of obese women. Int J Obes 1991;15(2):121–6.
7. Hauner H, Wabitsch M, Pfeiffer EF. Differentiation of adipocyte precursor cells from obese and non-obese adult women and from different adipose tissue sites. Horm Metab Res Suppl 1988;19: 35–9.
8. Billings E Jr, May JW Jr. Historical review and present status of free fat graft autotransplantation in plastic and reconstructive surgery. Plast Reconstr Surg 1989;83(2):368–81.
9. Katz AJ, Llull R, Hedrick MH, et al. Emerging approaches to the tissue engineering of fat. Clin Plast Surg 1999;26(4):587–603.
10. Patrick CW Jr, Chauvin PB, Hobley J, et al. Preadipocyte seeded PLGA scaffolds for adipose tissue engineering. Tissue Eng 1999;5(2):139–51.
11. Kimura Y, Ozeki M, Inamoto T, et al. Adipose tissue engineering based on human preadipocytes combined with gelatin microspheres containing basic fibroblast growth factor. Biomaterials 2003;24(14): 2513–21.
12. von Heimburg D, Kuberka M, Rendchen R, et al. Preadipocyte-loaded collagen scaffolds with enlarged pore size for improved soft tissue engineering. Int J Artif Organs 2003;26(12):1064–76.
13. Frye CA, Wu X, Patrick CW. Microvascular endothelial cells sustain preadipocyte viability under hypoxic conditions. In Vitro Cell Dev Biol Anim 2005;41(5–6):160–4.
14. Jarrell BE, Williams SK, Stokes G. Use of freshly isolated capillary endothelial cells for the immediate

establishment of a monolayer on a vascular graft at surgery. Surgery 1986;100(2):392–9.

15. Williams SK, Wang TF, Castrillo R, et al. Liposuction-derived human fat used for vascular graft sodding contains endothelial cells and not mesothelial cells as the major cell type. J Vasc Surg 1994;19(5):916–23.

16. Halvorsen YC, Wilkison WO, Gimble JM. Adipose-derived stromal cells–their utility and potential in bone formation. Int J Obes Relat Metab Disord 2000;24(Suppl 4):S41–4.

17. Zuk PA, Zhu M, Mizuno H, et al. Multilineage cells from human adipose tissue: implications for cell-based therapies. Tissue Eng 2001;7(2):211–28.

18. Crisan M, Yap S, Casteilla L, et al. A perivascular origin for mesenchymal stem cells in multiple human organs. Cell Stem Cell 2008;3(3):301–13.

19. Ergun S, Tilki D, Klein D. Vascular wall as a reservoir for different types of stem and progenitor cells. Antioxid Redox Signal 2011;15(4):981–95.

20. Zannettino AC, Paton S, Arthur A, et al. Multipotential human adipose-derived stromal stem cells exhibit a perivascular phenotype in vitro and in vivo. J Cell Physiol 2008;214(2):413–21.

21. Richardson RL, Hausman GJ, Campion DR. Response of pericytes to thermal lesion in the inguinal fat pad of 10-day-old rats. Acta Anat (Basel) 1982;114(1):41–57.

22. Hausman GJ, Campion DR, Martin RJ. Search for the adipocyte precursor cell and factors that promote its differentiation. J Lipid Res 1980;21(6):657–70.

23. Brighton CT, Hunt RM. Ultrastructure of electrically induced osteogenesis in the rabbit medullary canal. J Orthop Res 1986;4(1):27–36.

24. Brighton CT, Lorich DG, Kupcha R, et al. The pericyte as a possible osteoblast progenitor cell. Clin Orthop Relat Res 1992;(275):287–99.

25. Diaz-Flores L, Gutierrez R, Lopez-Alonso A, et al. Pericytes as a supplementary source of osteoblasts in periosteal osteogenesis. Clin Orthop Relat Res 1992;(275):280–6.

26. Silverman KJ, Lund DP, Zetter BR, et al. Angiogenic activity of adipose tissue. Biochem Biophys Res Commun 1988;153(1):347–52.

27. Hoying JB, Boswell CA, Williams SK. Angiogenic potential of microvessel fragments established in three-dimensional collagen gels. In Vitro Cell Dev Biol Anim 1996;32(7):409–19.

28. Crandall DL, Hausman GJ, Kral JG. A review of the microcirculation of adipose tissue: anatomic, metabolic, and angiogenic perspectives. Microcirculation 1997;4(2):211–32.

29. Bourin P, Bunnell BA, Casteilla L, et al. Stromal cells from the adipose tissue-derived stromal vascular fraction and culture expanded adipose tissue-derived stromal/stem cells: a joint statement of the International Federation for Adipose Therapeutics and Science (IFATS) and the International Society for Cellular Therapy (ISCT). Cytotherapy 2013;15(6):641–8.

30. Casteilla L, Planat-Benard V, Laharrague P, et al. Adipose-derived stromal cells: their identity and uses in clinical trials, an update. World J Stem Cells 2011;3(4):25–33.

31. Granel B, Daumas A, Jouve E, et al. Safety, tolerability and potential efficacy of injection of autologous adipose-derived stromal vascular fraction in the fingers of patients with systemic sclerosis: an open-label phase I trial. Ann Rheum Dis 2014. [Epub ahead of print].

32. Lee HC, An SG, Lee HW, et al. Safety and effect of adipose tissue-derived stem cell implantation in patients with critical limb ischemia: a pilot study. Circ J 2012;76(7):1750–60.

33. Park SA, Reilly CM, Wood JA, et al. Safety and immunomodulatory effects of allogeneic canine adipose-derived mesenchymal stromal cells transplanted into the region of the lacrimal gland, the gland of the third eyelid and the knee joint. Cytotherapy 2013;15(12):1498–510.

34. Ra JC, Shin IS, Kim SH, et al. Safety of intravenous infusion of human adipose tissue-derived mesenchymal stem cells in animals and humans. Stem Cells Dev 2011;20(8):1297–308.

35. Tzouvelekis A, Paspaliaris V, Koliakos G, et al. A prospective, non-randomized, no placebo-controlled, phase Ib clinical trial to study the safety of the adipose derived stromal cells-stromal vascular fraction in idiopathic pulmonary fibrosis. J Transl Med 2013;11:171.

36. Desai HV, Voruganti IS, Jayasuriya C, et al. Live-cell, temporal gene expression analysis of osteogenic differentiation in adipose-derived stem cells. Tissue Eng Part A 2013;19(1–2):40–8.

37. Hao W, Hu YY, Wei YY, et al. Collagen I gel can facilitate homogenous bone formation of adipose-derived stem cells in PLGA-beta-TCP scaffold. Cells Tissues Organs 2008;187(2):89–102.

38. Li X, Liu H, Niu X, et al. The use of carbon nanotubes to induce osteogenic differentiation of human adipose-derived MSCs in vitro and ectopic bone formation in vivo. Biomaterials 2012;33(19):4818–27.

39. Shi Y, Niedzinski JR, Samaniego A, et al. Adipose-derived stem cells combined with a demineralized cancellous bone substrate for bone regeneration. Tissue Eng Part A 2012;18(13–14):1313–21.

40. Yoon E, Dhar S, Chun DE, et al. In vivo osteogenic potential of human adipose-derived stem cells/poly lactide-co-glycolic acid constructs for bone regeneration in a rat critical-sized calvarial defect model. Tissue Eng 2007;13(3):619–27.

41. Chen Q, Yang Z, Sun S, et al. Adipose-derived stem cells modified genetically in vivo promote

reconstruction of bone defects. Cytotherapy 2010; 12(6):831–40.

42. Peterson B, Zhang J, Iglesias R, et al. Healing of critically sized femoral defects, using genetically modified mesenchymal stem cells from human adipose tissue. Tissue Eng 2005;11(1–2):120–9.

43. Zuk P. Adipose-derived stem cells in tissue regeneration: a review. Stem Cells 2013;2013:35.

44. Awad HA, Halvorsen YD, Gimble JM, et al. Effects of transforming growth factor beta1 and dexamethasone on the growth and chondrogenic differentiation of adipose-derived stromal cells. Tissue Eng 2003;9(6):1301–12.

45. Jin X, Sun Y, Zhang K, et al. Ectopic neocartilage formation from predifferentiated human adipose derived stem cells induced by adenoviral-mediated transfer of hTGF beta2. Biomaterials 2007;28(19):2994–3003.

46. Dragoo JL, Carlson G, McCormick F, et al. Healing full-thickness cartilage defects using adipose-derived stem cells. Tissue Eng 2007;13(7):1615–21.

47. Lu F, Gao JH, Ogawa R, et al. Adipose tissues differentiated by adipose-derived stem cells harvested from transgenic mice. Chin J Traumatol 2006;9(6):359–64.

48. Matsumoto D, Sato K, Gonda K, et al. Cell-assisted lipotransfer: supportive use of human adipose-derived cells for soft tissue augmentation with lipoinjection. Tissue Eng 2006;12(12):3375–82.

49. Eom YW, Lee JE, Yang MS, et al. Effective myotube formation in human adipose tissue-derived stem cells expressing dystrophin and myosin heavy chain by cellular fusion with mouse C2C12 myoblasts. Biochem Biophys Res Commun 2011; 408(1):167–73.

50. Choi YS, Vincent LG, Lee AR, et al. The alignment and fusion assembly of adipose-derived stem cells on mechanically patterned matrices. Biomaterials 2012;33(29):6943–51.

51. Wang C, Cen L, Yin S, et al. A small diameter elastic blood vessel wall prepared under pulsatile conditions from polyglycolic acid mesh and smooth muscle cells differentiated from adipose-derived stem cells. Biomaterials 2010; 31(4):621–30.

52. Heydarkhan-Hagvall S, Schenke-Layland K, Yang JQ, et al. Human adipose stem cells: a potential cell source for cardiovascular tissue engineering. Cells Tissues Organs 2008;187(4):263–74.

53. Vieira NM, Bueno CR Jr, Brandalise V, et al. SJL dystrophic mice express a significant amount of human muscle proteins following systemic delivery of human adipose-derived stromal cells without immunosuppression. Stem Cells 2008;26(9):2391–8.

54. Liu Y, Yan X, Sun Z, et al. Flk-1+ adipose-derived mesenchymal stem cells differentiate into skeletal muscle satellite cells and ameliorate muscular dystrophy in mdx mice. Stem Cells Dev 2007;16(5):695–706.

55. Zhao Z, Yu H, Xiao F, et al. Differentiation of adipose-derived stem cells promotes regeneration of smooth muscle for ureteral tissue engineering. J Surg Res 2012;178(1):55–62.

56. Zhang H, Qiu X, Shindel AW, et al. Adipose tissue-derived stem cells ameliorate diabetic bladder dysfunction in a type II diabetic rat model. Stem Cells Dev 2012;21(9):1391–400.

57. Otto Beitnes J, Oie E, Shahdadfar A, et al. Intramyocardial injections of human mesenchymal stem cells following acute myocardial infarction modulate scar formation and improve left ventricular function. Cell Transplant 2012;21(8):1697–709.

58. Yang J, Zhang H, Zhao L, et al. Human adipose tissue-derived stem cells protect impaired cardiomyocytes from hypoxia/reoxygenation injury through hypoxia-induced paracrine mechanism. Cell Biochem Funct 2012;30(6):505–14.

59. Yu JM, Bunnell BA, Kang SK. Neural differentiation of human adipose tissue-derived stem cells. Methods Mol Biol 2011;702:219–31.

60. Safford KM, Safford SD, Gimble JM, et al. Characterization of neuronal/glial differentiation of murine adipose-derived adult stromal cells. Exp Neurol 2004;187(2):319–28.

61. Leu S, Lin YC, Yuen CM, et al. Adipose-derived mesenchymal stem cells markedly attenuate brain infarct size and improve neurological function in rats. J Transl Med 2010;8:63.

62. Ryu HH, Lim JH, Byeon YE, et al. Functional recovery and neural differentiation after transplantation of allogenic adipose-derived stem cells in a canine model of acute spinal cord injury. J Vet Sci 2009; 10(4):273–84.

63. Wang Y, Zhao Z, Ren Z, et al. Recellularized nerve allografts with differentiated mesenchymal stem cells promote peripheral nerve regeneration. Neurosci Lett 2012;514(1):96–101.

64. Li H, Xu Y, Fu Q, et al. Effects of multiple agents on epithelial differentiation of rabbit adipose-derived stem cells in 3D culture. Tissue Eng Part A 2012; 18(17–18):1760–70.

65. Trottier V, Marceau-Fortier G, Germain L, et al. IFATS collection: using human adipose-derived stem/stromal cells for the production of new skin substitutes. Stem Cells 2008;26(10):2713–23.

66. Kim JM, Lee ST, Chu K, et al. Systemic transplantation of human adipose stem cells attenuated cerebral inflammation and degeneration in a hemorrhagic stroke model. Brain Res 2007;1183:43–50.

67. Cho KS, Roh HJ. Immunomodulatory effects of adipose-derived stem cells in airway allergic diseases. Curr Stem Cell Res Ther 2010;5(2):111–5.

68. Herreros MD, Garcia-Arranz M, Guadalajara H, et al. Autologous expanded adipose-derived stem cells for the treatment of complex cryptoglandular perianal fistulas: a phase III randomized clinical trial (FATT 1: fistula Advanced Therapy Trial 1) and long-term evaluation. Dis Colon Rectum 2012; 55(7):762–72.

69. Riordan NH, Ichim TE, Min WP, et al. Non-expanded adipose stromal vascular fraction cell therapy for multiple sclerosis. J Transl Med 2009; 7:29.

70. Ra JC, Kang SK, Shin IS, et al. Stem cell treatment for patients with autoimmune disease by systemic infusion of culture-expanded autologous adipose tissue derived mesenchymal stem cells. J Transl Med 2011;9:181.

71. Yanez R, Lamana ML, Garcia-Castro J, et al. Adipose tissue-derived mesenchymal stem cells have in vivo immunosuppressive properties applicable for the control of the graft-versus-host disease. Stem Cells 2006;24(11):2582–91.

72. Rehman J, Traktuev D, Li J, et al. Secretion of angiogenic and antiapoptotic factors by human adipose stromal cells. Circulation 2004;109(10): 1292–8.

73. Bayes-Genis A, Soler-Botija C, Farre J, et al. Human progenitor cells derived from cardiac adipose tissue ameliorate myocardial infarction in rodents. J Mol Cell Cardiol 2010;49(5):771–80.

74. DelaRosa O, Lombardo E, Beraza A, et al. Requirement of IFN-gamma-mediated indoleamine 2,3-dioxygenase expression in the modulation of lymphocyte proliferation by human adipose-derived stem cells. Tissue Eng Part A 2009; 15(10):2795–806.

75. Garcia-Olmo D, Garcia-Arranz M, Herreros D, et al. A phase I clinical trial of the treatment of Crohn's fistula by adipose mesenchymal stem cell transplantation. Dis Colon Rectum 2005;48(7):1416–23.

76. Garcia-Olmo D, Herreros D, Pascual I, et al. Expanded adipose-derived stem cells for the treatment of complex perianal fistula: a phase II clinical trial. Dis Colon Rectum 2009;52(1):79–86.

77. Kebriaei P, Robinson S. Treatment of graft-versus-host-disease with mesenchymal stromal cells. Cytotherapy 2011;13(3):262–8.

78. Moon KM, Park YH, Lee JS, et al. The effect of secretory factors of adipose-derived stem cells on human keratinocytes. Int J Mol Sci 2012;13(1): 1239–57.

79. Lee MJ, Kim J, Kim MY, et al. Proteomic analysis of tumor necrosis factor-alpha-induced secretome of human adipose tissue-derived mesenchymal stem cells. J Proteome Res 2010;9(4):1754–62.

80. Heo SC, Jeon ES, Lee IH, et al. Tumor necrosis factor-alpha-activated human adipose tissue-derived mesenchymal stem cells accelerate cutaneous wound healing through paracrine mechanisms. J Invest Dermatol 2011;131(7):1559–67.

81. Kapur SK, Katz AJ. Review of the adipose derived stem cell secretome. Biochimie 2013; 95(12):2222–8.

82. Marci L. Growth factor binding to the pericellular matrix and its importance in tissue engineering. Adv Drug Deliv Rev 2007;59:1366–81.

83. Clark RA. Synergistic signalling from extracellular matrix-growth factor complexes. J Invest Dermatol 2008;128:1354–5.

84. Amos PJ, Kapur SK, Stapor PC, et al. Human adipose-derived stromal cells accelerate diabetic wound healing: impact of cell formulation and delivery. Tissue Eng Part A 2010;16(5):1595–606.

85. Lin L, Fu X, Zhang X, et al. Rat adipose-derived stromal cells expressing BMP4 induce ectopic bone formation in vitro and in vivo. Acta Pharmacol Sin 2006;27(12):1608–15.

86. Josiah DT, Zhu D, Dreher F, et al. Adipose-derived stem cells as therapeutic delivery vehicles of an oncolytic virus for glioblastoma. Mol Ther 2010; 18(2):377–85.

87. Ning H, Lei HE, Xu YD, et al. Conversion of adipose-derived stem cells into natural killer-like cells with anti-tumor activities in nude mice. PLoS One 2014;9(8):e106246.

88. Aoki T, Ohnishi H, Oda Y, et al. Generation of induced pluripotent stem cells from human adipose-derived stem cells without c-MYC. Tissue Eng Part A 2010;16(7):2197–206.

89. Ohnishi H, Oda Y, Aoki T, et al. A comparative study of induced pluripotent stem cells generated from frozen, stocked bone marrow- and adipose tissue-derived mesenchymal stem cells. J Tissue Eng Regen Med 2012;6(4):261–71.

90. Gao Q, Zhao L, Song Z, et al. Expression pattern of embryonic stem cell markers in DFAT cells and ADSCs. Mol Biol Rep 2012;39(5):5791–804.

91. Nakagami H, Morishita R, Maeda K, et al. Adipose tissue-derived stromal cells as a novel option for regenerative cell therapy. J Atheroscler Thromb 2006;13(2):77–81.

92. Schaffler A, Buchler C. Concise review: adipose tissue-derived stromal cells–basic and clinical implications for novel cell-based therapies. Stem Cells 2007;25(4):818–27.

93. Bailey AM, Kapur S, Katz AJ. Characterization of adipose-derived stem cells: an update. Curr Stem Cell Res Ther 2010;5(2):95–102.

94. Senarath-Yapa K, McArdle A, Renda A, et al. Adipose-derived stem cells: a review of signaling networks governing cell fate and regenerative potential in the context of craniofacial and long bone skeletal repair. Int J Mol Sci 2014;15(6):9314–30.

95. Semon JA, Maness C, Zhang X, et al. Comparison of human adult stem cells from adipose tissue and

bone marrow in the treatment of experimental auto-immune encephalomyelitis. Stem Cell Res Ther 2014;5(1):2.

96. Marx C, Silveira MD, Selbach I, et al. Acupoint injection of autologous stromal vascular fraction and allogeneic adipose-derived stem cells to treat hip dysplasia in dogs. Stem Cells Int 2014;2014: 391274.

97. Jurgens WJ, Kroeze RJ, Zandieh-Doulabi B, et al. One-step surgical procedure for the treatment of osteochondral defects with adipose-derived stem cells in a caprine knee defect: a pilot study. Biores Open Access 2013;2(4):315–25.

98. Klopp AH, Gupta A, Spaeth E, et al. Concise review: dissecting a discrepancy in the literature: do mesenchymal stem cells support or suppress tumor growth? Stem Cells 2011;29(1):11–9.

99. Muehlberg FL, Song YH, Krohn A, et al. Tissue-resident stem cells promote breast cancer growth and metastasis. Carcinogenesis 2009;30(4): 589–97.

100. Yu JM, Jun ES, Bae YC, et al. Mesenchymal stem cells derived from human adipose tissues favor tumor cell growth in vivo. Stem Cells Dev 2008;17(3): 463–73.

101. Zimmerlin L, Donnenberg AD, Rubin JP, et al. Regenerative therapy and cancer: in vitro and in vivo studies of the interaction between adipose-derived stem cells and breast cancer cells from clinical isolates. Tissue Eng Part A 2011; 17(1–2):93–106.

102. Zhang Y, Daquinag A, Traktuev DO, et al. White adipose tissue cells are recruited by experimental tumors and promote cancer progression in mouse models. Cancer Res 2009;69(12):5259–66.

103. Linkov F, Kokai L, Edwards R, et al. The role of adipose-derived stem cells in endometrial cancer proliferation. Scand J Clin Lab Invest Suppl 2014; 244:54–8 [discussion: 57–8].

104. Kuhbier JW, Bucan V, Reimers K, et al. Observed changes in the morphology and phenotype of breast cancer cells in direct co-culture with adipose-derived stem cells. Plast Reconstr Surg 2014;134(3):414–23.

105. Zhu Y, Sun Z, Han Q, et al. Human mesenchymal stem cells inhibit cancer cell proliferation by secreting DKK-1. Leukemia 2009;23(5):925–33.

106. Qiao L, Xu ZL, Zhao TJ, et al. Dkk-1 secreted by mesenchymal stem cells inhibits growth of breast cancer cells via depression of Wnt signalling. Cancer Lett 2008;269(1):67–77.

107. Sun B, Roh KH, Park JR, et al. Therapeutic potential of mesenchymal stromal cells in a mouse breast cancer metastasis model. Cytotherapy 2009;11(3): 289–98.

108. Cousin B, Ravet E, Poglio S, et al. Adult stromal cells derived from human adipose tissue provoke pancreatic cancer cell death both in vitro and in vivo. PLoS One 2009;4(7):e6278.

109. Perez-Cano R, Vranckx JJ, Lasso JM, et al. Prospective trial of adipose-derived regenerative cell (ADRC)-enriched fat grafting for partial mastectomy defects: the RESTORE-2 trial. Eur J Surg Oncol 2012;38(5):382–9.

110. Gronthos S, Franklin DM, Leddy HA, et al. Surface protein characterization of human adipose tissue-derived stromal cells. Journal of cellular physiology 2001;189:54–63.

111. Zuk PA, Zhu M, Ashjian P, et al. Human adipose tissue is a source of multipotent stem cells. Molecular biology of the cell 2002;13:4279–95.

112. Katz AJ, Tholpady A, Tholpady SS, et al. Cell surface and transcriptional characterization of human adipose-derived adherent stromal (hADAS) cells. Stem Cells 2005;23:412–23.

113. Mitchell JB, McIntosh K, Zvonic S, et al. Immunophenotype of human adipose-derived cells: temporal changes in stromal-associated and stem cell-associated markers. Stem Cells 2006;24:376–85.

114. Yoshimura K, Shigeura T, Matsumoto D, et al. Characterization of freshly isolated and cultured cells derived from the fatty and fluid portions of liposuction aspirates. Journal of cellular physiology 2006; 208:64–76.

115. Varma MJ, Breuls RG, Schouten TE, et al. Phenotypical and functional characterization of freshly isolated adipose tissue-derived stem cells. Stem cells and development 2007;16:91–104.

116. Traktuev DO, Merfeld-Clauss S, Li J, et al. A population of multipotent CD34-positive adipose stromal cells share pericyte and mesenchymal surface markers, reside in a periendothelial location, and stabilize endothelial networks. Circulation research 2008;102:77–85.

117. Zimmerlin L, Donnenberg VS, Pfeifer ME, et al. Stromal vascular progenitors in adult human adipose tissue. Cytometry Part A. the journal of the International Society for Analytical Cytology 2010;77: 22–30.

118. Lin G, Garcia M, Ning H, et al. Defining stem and progenitor cells within adipose tissue. Stem cells and development 2008;17:1053–63.

Adipose Stem Cells
Biology, Safety, Regulation, and Regenerative Potential

Danielle M. Minteer, BS[a], Kacey G. Marra, PhD[a,b,c],
J. Peter Rubin, MD[a,b,c],*

KEYWORDS

- Adipose • Adipose-derived stem cells • Tissue engineering • Regenerative medicine
- Clinical translation • Mesenchymal stem cells • Stromal vascular fraction • Stem cell safety

KEY POINTS

- Human adipose tissue is now a widely accepted source for stem cells in regenerative medicine, and has been the subject of preclinical studies and clinical studies directed toward numerous applications.
- The nonlipid cell population isolated from adipose tissue is heterogeneous and contains adipose-derived stem cells (ASCs), which can be isolated and cultured.
- ASCs are of mesenchymal lineage and manifest features that are attractive for regenerative therapy approaches, including multipotency and release of growth factors that can induce tissue healing.
- These beneficial characteristics have the potential to affect cancer growth and this issue is still being investigated in preclinical and clinical studies.
- From a regulatory perspective, adipose therapies may be regulated under the category of human cells, tissues, and cellular and tissue-based products by the US Food and Drug Administration in Title 21 Code of Federal Regulations, part 1271, or as a biologic drug under section 351 of the Public Health Services Act, depending on the specific use and the degree of processing.
- To date, 129 active clinical trials are listed in the US National Institutes of Health Web site (www.clinicaltrials.gov), spanning a broad range of applications including arthritis, intervertebral disc degeneration, autism therapy, cell-enriched fat grafting, pulmonary disease, and numerous clinical targets.

ISOLATION AND CHARACTERIZATION

Adipose-derived stem cells (ASCs) are prevalent surrounding the blood vessels and within the connective tissue of human adipose tissue. These non–lipid-laden stromal cells can be isolated from either suction-aspirated adipose tissue or excised human fat by enzymatic collagenase digestion. Passenger erythrocytes can be lysed selectively, and numerous descriptions for cell isolation methods appear in the literature.[1–3] The freshly isolated cell pellet is highly heterogeneous and is named the stromal vascular fraction (SVF). Further discussion of the SVF components is featured later. If the SVF cells are placed in culture, the ASCs adhere to the surface of an untreated tissue culture flask after 6 to 8 hours' incubation at 37°C and 5% CO_2. Once ASCs have adhered to the culture flask surface, nonadherent

[a] Department of Bioengineering, University of Pittsburgh, 200 Lothrop Street, Pittsburgh, PA 15213, USA;
[b] Department of Plastic Surgery, University of Pittsburgh, 3550 Terrace Street, Pittsburgh, PA 15213, USA;
[c] McGowan Institute for Regenerative Medicine, University of Pittsburgh, 450 Technology Drive, Pittsburgh, PA 15213, USA
* Corresponding author. Department of Plastic Surgery, University of Pittsburgh, 3550 Terrace Street, Pittsburgh, PA 15213.
E-mail address: rubipj@upmc.edu

Clin Plastic Surg 42 (2015) 169–179
http://dx.doi.org/10.1016/j.cps.2014.12.007

populations, representing 7% to 15% of the SVF and representing mainly hematopoietic origin cells, are washed away with sterile phosphate buffered solution and/or fresh culture media. **Fig. 1** shows a widely accepted protocol for SVF and ASC isolation.[4] A commonly used ASC expansion medium consists of a Dulbecco's Modified Eagle Medium (DMEM) and DMEM/F12 media combination, with 10% serum, antibiotic (eg, penicillin, streptomycin), and a small amount of dexamethasone to prevent differentiation to another mesenchymal lineage. Once in culture, specific growth factors or other additives can be applied to direct the differentiation to a specific phenotype, such as adipose, bone, cartilage, or muscle.

SVF is attractive therapeutically because it may be obtained from tissue within 60 to 90 minutes, and the isolation can be performed in a clean room near an operating room, or even in an operating room using an automated device. Collagenase digestion results in approximately 2×10^5 to 5×10^5 nucleated SVF cells per gram of adipose tissue. However, the complete ASC isolation process takes 20 to 24 hours and requires cell culture facilities. Reasons to culture the cells include the ability to expand the cell number, select for specific subpopulation, or control the microenvironment for directed differentiation or induction of

adherence to a scaffold material. Flow cytometry characterization of the surface markers on freshly isolated and cultured adipose-derived cells can be performed, and shows the presence of early progenitor markers such as cluster of differentiation 34 (CD34) and CD90.[4,5]

Nonenzymatic cell isolation has been a topic of interest, driven by a potentially less restrictive regulatory pathway. This strategy has focused on mechanical forces such as ultrasound. However, there is no strong evidence to suggest that this is equivalent to enzymatic digestion. There has also been interest in whether there are viable ASCs in the aqueous portion of the liposuction aspirate without exposure of the tissue to enzymes. Although some cells may be present, the quantity is so low as to preclude clinical utility. Because the ASCs are firmly embedded within the connective tissue, enzymatic digestion is necessary to release them in significant quantity.

Preadipocytes were first described in 1976 by Dardick and colleagues,[6] beginning with rat models then isolated from human tissues.[7-9] Isolated preadipocytes were used to study adipocyte biology in vitro, leading to recognition of different anatomic locations and adipose depots to express different biological characteristics, such as adipocyte size and lipolytic potential. In 2001, Zuk and colleagues[10] first discussed the differentiation

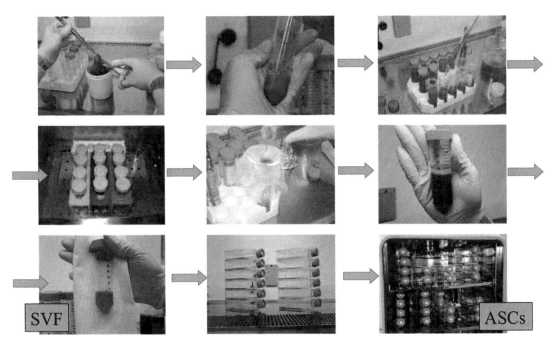

Fig. 1. The SVF and ASC isolation process as described by Rubin and Marra.[4] First, whole adipose tissue or lipoaspirate is finely minced and enzyme digested in at 37°C. Red blood cells are lysed and the suspension is filtered. Following centrifugation, the pellet is considered the SVF. Once plated and cultured on a tissue culture flask at 37°C and 5% CO_2 for 6 to 8 hours, the mesenchymal ASCs are obtained. (*Adapted from* Rubin JP, Marra KG. Soft tissue reconstruction. Methods Mol Biol 2011;702:397; with permission.)

plasticity of preadipocytes and eventually the term ASC was adopted to encompass the characteristics of self-renewal, asymmetric division, and multipotency. Although ASCs proliferate rapidly in culture in vivo, growth factors are necessary to induce lineage-specific differentiation.[4] Differentiation of ASCs to other mesenchymal phenotypes has been well established both in vitro and in vivo. ASC differentiation to cell lineages of the ectodermal and endodermal germ layers has also been successful in several studies.[11–30] Gerlach and colleagues[17] described adipogenesis

within a hollow fiber–based, three-dimensional, dynamic perfusion bioreactor in which ASCs are differentiated and maintained as functional, mature adipocytes long term (**Fig. 2**).

The SVF population (the freshly isolated population) derived from adipose tissue has diverse patterns of cell surface markers as identified by flow cytometry.[5,14] Zimmerlin and colleagues[5] identified several similar cell surface markers in ASCs (the cultured population) compared with bone marrow–derived stem cells (BMSCs) and these are described in **Table 1**. Li and colleagues[2]

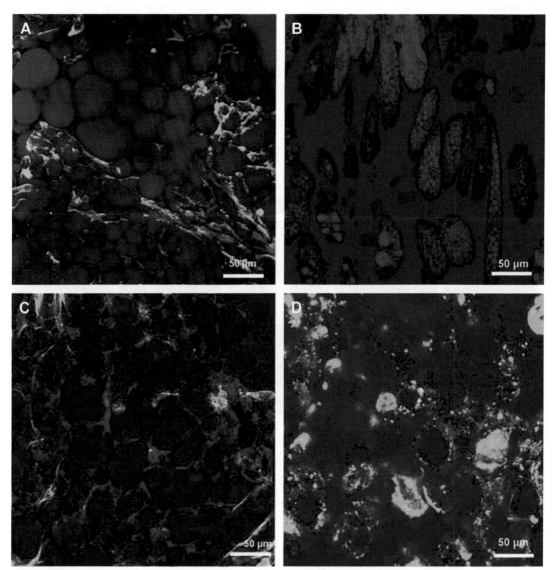

Fig. 2. Confocal microscopy of adipose tissue generated within hollow fiber–based, three-dimensional, dynamic perfusion bioreactors (*A*, *C*) and the two-dimensional control treatment (*B*, *D*).[17] Samples were stained with 4′,6-Diamidino-2-Phenylindole, Dihydrochloride (DAPI) (*blue*), Alexa Fluor® 488 for phalloidin (*green*), and the following fluorescent markers using cyanine dye 3 (Cy3) (*red*): (*A, B*) AdipoRed™, (*C, D*) glucose transporter 4. (*From* Gerlach JC, Lin YC, Brayfield CA, et al. Adipogenesis of human adipose-derived stem cells within three-dimensional hollow fiber-based bioreactors. Tissue Eng 2012;18(1):58; with permission.)

Table 1
Surface marker characterization of ASCs and BMSCs

	ASCs	BMSCs
Negative	CD38, CD45, CD106, HLA-DR, DP, DQ (MHC class II), CD80, CD86, CD40, and CD40L (CD154)	CD34, CD38, CD45, and fox antigens involved in immunologic signal transduction such as HLA-DR, DP, DQ (MHC class II), CD80, CD86, CD40, and CD40L (CD154)
Positive	CD13, CD29, CD34, CD44, CD73, CD90, CD105, CD166, MHC class I, HLA-ABC	CD13, CD29, CD44, CD73, CD90, CD105, CD166, MHC class I, HLA-ABC

ASCs were freshly isolated and examined via flow cytometry.
(*Adapted from* Minteer D, Marra KG, Rubin J. Adipose derived mesenchymal stem cells: biology and potential applications. Mesenchymal stem cells basics and clinical application I. Berlin Heidelberg: Springer; 2013. p. 59–71.)

reported 4 subpopulations of interest that can be isolated and cultured (**Fig. 3**). The first is CD31+/34-, which is classified as mature endothelial, with the endothelial marker of CD31, lacking the progenitor marker of CD34. The second subpopulation is classified as "endothelial stem," and CD31+/34+. A third subpopulation, CD34+/31- is classified as the adipose stem cell group.

The fourth subpopulation represents a pericyte group and is characterized by surface markers CD146+/90+/31-/34-. These cells reside adjacent to the blood vessel walls, and are shown by immunostaining.[15] Similar to BMSCs, ASCs do not express major histocompatibility complex (MHC)-II and inhibit proliferation of activated peripheral blood mononuclear cells, suggesting a role for

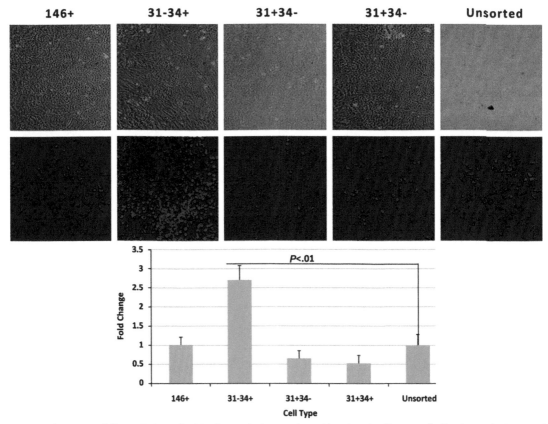

Fig. 3. Adipogenic differentiation of ASC subpopulations as found by Li and colleagues.[2] All subpopulations and unsorted cells were exposed to adipogenic differentiation medium for 2 weeks; AdipoRed™ determined lipid accumulation via fluorescence microscopy and quantification. (*From* Li H, Zimmerlin L, Marra KG, et al. Adipogenic potential of adipose stem cell subpopulations. Plast Reconstr Surg 2011;128(3):669; with permission.)

modulating the immune system in inflammatory disorders or allogeneic transplantation.[14]

USE OF ADIPOSE-DERIVED STEM CELLS TO ENHANCE FAT GRAFTING

To improve results in fat transfer, a clinical strategy has been developed in which autologous SVF cells are admixed with the fat graft to promote graft volume retention and neovascularization.[31–34] Named cell-assisted lipotransfer (CAL), the appeal of ASC incorporation in lipoinjection is mostly because of growth factor release of the stem cells, especially angiogenic growth factors such as vascular endothelial growth factor. Another hypothesis supporting ASC addition to the fat graft includes the concept that ASCs provide a scaffold on which additional stem cells can organize and differentiate. This strategy has further appeal because the SVF can be isolated at the point of care.

The first randomized controlled study to show the efficacy of this strategy in humans was published in 2013 by Kølle and colleagues.[35] Human volunteers received 2 fat grafts, one in each upper extremity, both with and without supplemental stem cells. The grafts admixed with stem cells showed significantly higher volume retention. This study provided proof of principle in a clinical trial, but had several notable criticisms. First, the cell dose was exceedingly high, with 2×10^7 cells admixed with each milliliter of fat injected. Second, the ability to obtain such a high cell dose required expansion of the harvested SVF in cell culture, which involves high cost and regulatory hurdles beyond the use of SVF alone. In addition, culturing cells requires a separate fat harvest procedure. Third, the fat graft was administered as a 30-cm^3 bolus injection, rather than as a fanning technique that disperses the fat graft within the recipient bed.[36] The concept of CAL is being used for aesthetic and reconstructive applications across the body. The question of cell dose, or the minimum quantity of nucleated SVF cells that needs to be added to each milliliter of graft for clinical effect, remains an area of study.

INTERACTIONS BETWEEN ADIPOSE-DERIVED STEM CELLS AND TUMOR CELLS

The same properties of that make ASCs useful for tissue healing and regeneration also create the potential for the stimulation of tumor cell growth when the cells are used for cancer reconstruction.[37] Characteristics frequently shared between tumor progression and successful regenerative therapies intended to restore functional tissue include cellular homing, immunosuppression, revascularization, and tissue growth promotion.[38]

In addition to the direct secretion of angiogenic growth factors, which could induce a nourishing vascular supply to tumors, ASCs secrete large quantities of leptin and adipsin.[39] Leptin increases angiogenic and proliferative signaling in estrogen receptor–positive and estrogen receptor–negative breast cancer cell lines.[40] Adipsin has been proved to increase the concentration of acylation-stimulating protein, which is another adipose-derived hormone that regulates triglyceride synthesis.[41]

Zimmerlin and colleagues[38] reviewed the mesenchymal stem cell (MSC) secretome and regenerative therapy after cancer, outlining direct and indirect secretome properties in connection with MSC paracrine effects and differentiation, and summarized MSC–tumor cell interactions. These properties were not known when autologous fat grafting was first pioneered at the end of the nineteenth century.[42,43]

With an in vitro coculture model, Zimmerlin and colleagues[44] confirmed an enhancing effect of ASCs on the proliferation of breast cancer cells (proliferating but not dormant cells), confirming the results of several other studies proving MSC presence can stimulate tumor cell growth.[45–47] In addition, more evidence has accumulated suggesting that clonogenic tumor cells share many characteristics with adult tissue stem cells, including self-renewal.[48–50]

In their review article analyzing risks of regenerative therapy after cancer, Donnenberg and colleagues[37] distinguished between 2 potentially tumorigenic populations, resting (dormant) and active (proliferating) tumor cells, and the parallels that may be associated with adult tissue stem cells. They hypothesized that the driving stimuli pushing dormant stem–like cancer cells into an active tumorigenic state are distinct from the stimuli that favor the survival and proliferation of active progenitorlike tumor cells. Such a hypothesis guides the concept that introducing proangiogenic autologous MSCs after tumor resection when the region is clinically disease free would not contribute to local recurrence and, if increased local vascularization at the tumor site was an independent risk factor for recurrence, it would become more clear after observing patients reconstructed with well-vascularized tissue flaps. Immediate autologous tissue flap reconstruction has not been associated with heightened recurrence rates.[51] Therefore, stem cell–based therapies for reconstruction after cancer would be safe if the patient is clinically disease free.

Although in vitro studies suggest that ASCs stimulate tumor growth, the situation of high concentrations of stem cells in close proximity with tumor cells ex vivo may not accurately model the clinical scenario of CAL for breast reconstruction, and the clinical significance of these studies remains unclear. The question will best be answered in large clinical trials. To date, large patient series of autologous fat transfer for breast reconstruction, representing the application of both adipocytes and native adipose stem cells to a tumor bed, show either no increased rate of recurrence or a relationship only in a subgroup of young patients with highly aggressive tumors.[52,53]

REGULATION OF ADIPOSE STEM CELLS

Regulation of ASC exploration varies based on nation. In the European Union, the European Medicines Agency oversees such studies, as does the Pharmaceutical and Medical Devices Agency in Japan. In the United States, the Center for Biologics Evaluation and Research sector within the US Food and Drug Administration (FDA) has authority over stem cell products.

In the United States, ASCs can be considered human cells, tissues, and cellular product and tissue-based products (HCT/Ps) by the FDA and may potentially be regulated under section 361 of the Public Health Service (PHS) Act (42 U.S.C. 264).[54,55]

Regulation 21 CFR 1271 details what procedures should be established and maintained in testing, screening, determining donor eligibility, and complying with all other requirements as well as approved shipping and storage information of HCT/Ps in order to prevent the spread of communicable diseases.[54] In order for a cell or tissue product to be classified under this regulation, it must be applied for homologous use and the cells and tissues must be minimally manipulated. However, there is debate over whether the enzymatic digestion used to isolate the ASCs constitutes more than minimal manipulation of the tissue and places the cell product into the category of a biologic drug as defined in section 351(i) of the PHS Act (42 U.S.C. 262(i)). The implications for this classification are significant. A cell therapy regulated as an HCT/P requires adherence to strict manufacturing guidelines. In contrast, a therapy regulated as a biologic product must be tested for efficacy and safety in phase 1, 2, and 3 clinical trials, and then be granted a biologic license.

REGENERATIVE POTENTIAL OF ADIPOSE-DERIVED STEM CELLS

Although soft tissue regeneration has been a prominent clinical target for ASC therapies in plastic and reconstructive surgery, a wide range of applications exist. Because ASCs isolated from human adipose tissue have high potential for differentiation into mature adipocytes and other tissue types along the mesenchyme lineage, including chondrocytes, osteoblasts, and skeletal and cardiac muscle, numerous disease processes can be addressed.[6,11,14–17]

There is much interest in whether gender influences ASC biology, and the impact of gender and anatomic region on osteogenic differentiation of ASCs has been evaluated in vitro.[56] ASCs isolated from the superficial and deep adipose layers of male and female patients were exposed to osteogenic differentiation medium for periods of 1, 2, and 4 weeks. Through alkaline phosphatase, alizarin red, and Masson trichrome staining, as well as enzyme-linked immunosorbent assay and Western blot analysis, the group was able to determine that no significant difference in the amount of osteogenic differentiation exists in both fat depots from women, whereas the superficial depot in men provided ASCs that differentiated sooner and more efficiently than ASCs from the deep fat depots. Furthermore, it was established that male ASCs differentiated more effectively into osteoblasts than female ASCs from all depots.

In studying the regenerative potential of ASCs, many investigations involve defined culture conditions and techniques.[3,57,58] To address large-scale culture experiments examining adipogenesis, the 3T3-L1 cell mouse line proves a useful model when consistency of cells is required over time. Cells from the 3T3-L1 line are easily differentiated into adipocytes under the appropriate conditions in vitro.[16] For long-term culture experiments, bioreactor systems that are composed of three-dimensional culture chambers with the ability to perfuse nutrient media and carefully control all aspects of the microenvironment are an excellent tool for studying ASC biology. These systems not only serve as models for engineering tissues but also show the metabolic parameters of a self-contained, ex vivo organ system and can be used as a drug discovery tool.[17,57,59]

To date, 129 active clinical trials are listed in the US National Institutes of Health Web site (clinicaltrials.gov), spanning a broad range of applications. As well as soft tissue regeneration, other applications of ASC regenerative potential exist around skeletal tissue repair[29,60–66]; ischemic injuries and myocardial infarction[19,67–79]; gene therapy[80–84]; and immune disorders such as lupus, arthritis, colitis, Crohn disease, multiple sclerosis, diabetes mellitus, and graft-versus-host disease.[85–112] Treatment of chronic or otherwise difficult-to-heal wounds is being aggressively pursued. The cells can be injected into the wound bed or applied topically. A recently validated strategy using ASCs delivered via a fibrin spray vehicle has been described.[44] Other targets being explored in clinical trials include intervertebral disc degeneration, autism, and pulmonary disease.[111]

Academic institutions, academic hospitals, governmental funding agencies, private biotechnology corporations, and others are using ASCs in studies.[113] It is important to acknowledge that, as clinical translation and applications of ASCs continue to expand, validation and compliance of good manufacturing practice (GMP) guidelines are equally crucial. To ensure quality, a laboratory must reduce risk of contamination, define the in-process and lot-release criteria, and conduct functional assays and sterility testing of the ASCs.[113–116]

In 2002, the US National Heart, Lung, and Blood Institute hosted a workshop to address the needs of the cell therapy community. From this workshop emerged a contract consisting of 3 cell-manufacturing facilities and 1 administrative center to provide manufacturing resources, improved access to GMP facilities, regulatory assistance, and training to foster the advancement of cellular therapy.[117] As of 2009, in a 5-year report, the Production Assistance for Cellular Therapies (PACT) announced submission of 65 preliminary applications from 55 different investigators requesting manufacturing support for cellular therapy products. Forty were external (PACT includes Baylor College of Medicine, University of Minnesota, University of Pittsburgh, and the EMMES Corporation), 19 were from a non-PACT investigator at a PACT site, and 6 were internal applications from PACT investigators. Within PACT's listing of cell therapy product requests and treatment indications were MSCs, ASCs, and autologous CD34+ stem cells to treat cardiac damage in patients after myocardial infarction, sickle cell disease, and ischemia and intermittent claudication, respectively.[117] The University of Pittsburgh ASC clinical protocols were developed with PACT funding.

SUMMARY

ASCs remain an important source of multipotent cells, with their abundance and ease of access making ASCs a popular choice in modern tissue engineering strategies. To ensure validated technological advancement of ASC studies, cooperation with and involvement of GMP facilities is necessary. ASCs are a promising source of autologous stem cells for numerous tissue engineering and regenerative medicine applications.

REFERENCES

1. Ando H, Yanagihara H, Hayashi Y, et al. Rhythmic messenger ribonucleic acid expression of clock genes and adipocytokines in mouse visceral adipose tissue. Endocrinology 2005;146(12):5631–6.
2. Li H, Zimmerlin L, Marra KG, et al. Adipogenic potential of adipose stem cell subpopulations. Plast Reconstr Surg 2011;128(3):663–72.
3. Minteer D, Marra KG, Peter Rubin J. Adipose-derived mesenchymal stem cells: biology and potential applications. Mesenchymal stem cells-basics and clinical application I. Berlin, Heidelberg: Springer; 2013. p. 59–71.
4. Rubin JP, Marra KG. Soft tissue reconstruction. Methods Mol Biol 2011;702:395–400.
5. Zimmerlin L, Donnenberg VS, Pfeifer ME, et al. Stromal vascular progenitors in adult human adipose tissue. Cytometry A 2010;77(1):22–30.
6. Dardick I, Poznanski WJ, Waheed I, et al. Ultrastructural observations on differentiating human preadipocytes cultured in vitro. Tissue Cell 1976; 8(3):561–71.
7. Emre Aksu A, Rubin JP, Dudas JR, et al. Role of gender and anatomical region on induction of osteogenic differentiation of human adipose-derived stem cells. Ann Plast Surg 2008;60(3):306–20.
8. Green H, Kehinde O. An established preadipose cell line and its differentiation in culture II. Factors affecting the adipose conversion. Cell 1975;5(1): 19–27.
9. Hollenberg CH, Vost A. Regulation of DNA synthesis in fat cells and stromal elements from rat adipose tissue. J Clin Invest 1968;47:2485–98.
10. Zuk PA, Zhu M, Mizuno H, et al. Multilineage cells from human adipose tissue: implications for cell-based therapies. Tissue Eng 2001;7(2):211–28.
11. Stiles JW, Francendese AA, Masoro EJ. Influence of age on size and number of fat cells in the epididymal depot. Am J Physiol 1975;229(6):1561–8.
12. Mehlhorn AT, Niemeyer P, Kaiser S, et al. Differential expression pattern of extracellular matrix molecules during chondrogenesis of mesenchymal stem cells from bone marrow and adipose tissue. Tissue Eng 2006;12(10):2853–62.
13. Planat-Bénard V, Menard C, André C, et al. Spontaneous cardiomyocyte differentiation from adipose tissue stroma cells. Circ Res 2004;94:223–9.
14. Brayfield CA, Marra KG, Rubin JP. Adipose stem cells for soft tissue regeneration. Handchir Mikrochir Plast Chir 2010;42:124–8.
15. Bunnell BA, Estes BT, Guilak F, et al. Differentiation of adipose stem cells. Methods Mol Biol 2008;456: 155–71.
16. Frye CA, Patrick CW. Three-dimensional adipose tissue model using low shear bioreactor. In Vitro Cell Dev Biol Anim 2006;42(5):109–14.

17. Gerlach JC, Lin YC, Brayfield CA, et al. Adipogenesis of human adipose-derived stem cells within three-dimensional hollow fiber-based bioreactors. Tissue Eng 2012;18(1):54–61.

18. Zuk PA, Zhu M, Ashjian P, et al. Human adipose tissue is a source of multipotent stem cells. Mol Biol Cell 2002;13(12):4279–95.

19. Miyahara Y, Nagaya N, Kataoka K, et al. Monolayered mesenchymal stem cells repair scarred myocardium after myocardial infarction. Nat Med 2006;12(4):459–65.

20. Strem BM, Hicok KC, Zhu M, et al. Multipotential differentiation of adipose tissue-derived stem cells. Keio J Med 2005;54(3):132–41.

21. Choi YS, Cha SM, Lee YY, et al. Adipogenic differentiation of adipose tissue derived adult stem cells in nude mouse. Biochem Biophys Res Commun 2006;345(2):631–7.

22. Kimura Y, Ozeki M, Inamoto T, et al. Adipose tissue engineering based on human preadipocytes combined with gelatin microspheres containing basic fibroblast growth factor. Biomaterials 2003;24:2513–21.

23. Lee JH, Kemp DM. Human adipose-derived stem cells display myogenic potential and perturbed function in hypoxic conditions. Biochem Biophys Res Commun 2006;341(3):882–8.

24. Rodriguez LV, Alfonso ZC, Zhang R, et al. Clonogenic multipotent stem cells in human adipose tissue differentiate in muscle cells. Proc Natl Acad Sci U S A 2006;103(32):12167–72.

25. Gaustad KG, Boquest AC, Anderson BE, et al. Differentiation of human adipose tissue stem cells using extracts of rat cardiomyocytes. Biochem Biophys Res Commun 2004;314(2):420–7.

26. Miranville A, Heeschen C, Sengenés C, et al. Development of postnatal neovascularization by human adipose tissue-derived stem cells. Circulation 2004;110:349–55.

27. Lin Y, Chen X, Yan Z, et al. Multilineage differentiation of adipose-derived stromal cells from GFP transgenic mice. Mol Cell Biochem 2006;285(1–2):69–78.

28. Ning H, Lin G, Lue TF, et al. Neuron-like differentiation of adipose tissue-derived stromal cells and vascular smooth muscle cells. Differentiation 2006;74(9–10):510–8.

29. Cowan CM, Aalami OO, Shi YY, et al. Bone morphogenetic protein 2 and retinoic acid accelerate in vivo bone formation, osteoclast recruitment, and bone turnover. Tissue Eng 2005;11(3–4):645–58.

30. Kang SK, Lee DH, Bae YC, et al. Improvement of neurological deficits by intracerebral transplantation of human adipose tissue-derived stromal cells after cerebral ischemia in rats. Exp Neurol 2003;183(2):355–66.

31. Yoshimura K, Sato K, Aoi N, et al. Cell-assisted lipotransfer for facial lipoatrophy: efficacy of clinical use of adipose-derived stem cells. Dermatol Surg 2008;34:1178.

32. Yoshimura K, Sato K, Aoi N, et al. Cell-assisted lipotransfer for cosmetic breast augmentation: supportive use of adipose-derived stem/stromal cells. Aesthetic Plast Surg 2008;32:48 [discussion: 6–7].

33. Matsumoto D, Sato K, Gonda K, et al. Cell-assisted lipotransfer: supportive use of human adipose-derived cells for soft tissue augmentation with lipoinjection. Tissue Eng 2006;12:3375.

34. Moseley TA, Zhu M, Hedrick MH. Adipose-derived stem and progenitor cells as fillers in plastic and reconstructive surgery. Plast Reconstr Surg 2006;118:121S.

35. Kølle SF, Fischer-Nielsen A, Mathiasen AB, et al. Enrichment of autologous fat grafts with ex-vivo expanded adipose tissue-derived stem cells for graft survival: a randomised placebo-controlled trial. Lancet 2013;382(9898):1113–20.

36. Rubin JP, Marra KG. Commentary. Cell-assisted lipotransfer (CAL). Aesthet Surg J 2010;30:82.

37. Donnenberg VS, Zimmerlin L, Rubin JP, et al. Regenerative therapy after cancer: what are the risks? Tissue Eng Part B Rev 2010;16(6):567–75.

38. Zimmerlin L, Park TS, Zambidis ET, et al. Mesenchymal stem cell secretome and regenerative therapy after cancer. Biochimie 2013;95(12):2235–45.

39. Zimmerlin L, Donnenberg AD, Rubin JP, et al. Regenerative therapy and cancer: in vitro and in vivo studies of the interaction between adipose-derived stem cells and breast cancer cells from clinical isolates. Tissue Eng Part A 2011;17:93–106.

40. Rene Gonzalez R, Watters A, Xu Y, et al. Leptin-signaling inhibition results in efficient anti-tumor activity in estrogen receptor positive or negative breast cancer. Breast Cancer Res 2009;11:R36.

41. Baldo A, Sniderman AD, St. Luce S, et al. The adipsin-acylation stimulating protein system and regulation of intracellular triglyceride synthesis. J Clin Invest 1993;92:1543.

42. Neuber F. Fettransplantation. Verh Dtsch Ges Chir 22(1893):66.

43. Czerny M. Reconstruction of the breast with a lipoma. Chir Kongr Verh 2 (1895): 216.

44. Zimmerlin L, Rubin JP, Pfeifer ME, et al. Human adipose stromal vascular cell delivery in a fibrin spray. Cytotherapy 2012;15:102–8.

45. Pinilla S, Alt E, Abdul Khalek FJ, et al. Tissue resident stem cells produce CCL5 under the influence of cancer cells and thereby promote breast cancer cell invasion. Cancer Lett 2009;284:80.

46. Kucerova L, Matuskova M, Hlubinova K, et al. Tumor cell behaviour modulation by mesenchymal stromal cells. Mol Cancer 2010;9:129.

47. Almog N, Ma L, Raychowdhury R, et al. Transcriptional switch of dormant tumors to fast-growing angiogenic phenotype. Cancer Res 2009;69:836.

48. Donnenberg VS, Luketich JD, Landreneau RJ, et al. Tumorigenic epithelial stem cells and their normal counterparts. Ernst Schering Found Symp Proc 2006;5:245.

49. Abraham BK, Fritz P, McClellan M, et al. Prevalence of CD44+/CD24-/low cells in breast cancer may not be associated with clinical outcome but may favor distant metastasis. Clin Cancer Res 2005; 11:1154.

50. Sheridan C, Kishimoto H, Fuchs RK, et al. CD44+/CD24- breast cancer cells exhibit enhanced invasive properties: an early step necessary for metastasis. Breast Cancer Res 2006;8:R59.

51. Min SY, Kim HY, Jung SY, et al. Oncological safety and quality of life associated with mastectomy and immediate breast construction with a latissimus dorsi myocutaneous flap. Breast J 2010;16:356.

52. Delay E, Garson S, Tousson G, et al. Fat injection to the breast: technique, results, and indications based on 880 procedures over 10 years. Aesthet Surg J 2009;29:360.

53. Petit JY, Botteri E, Lohsiriwat V, et al. Locoregional recurrence risk after lipofilling in breast cancer patients. Ann Oncol 2012;23(3):582–8.

54. Eligibility determination for donors of human cells, tissues, and cellular and tissue-based products (HCT/Ps). 21 CFR 1271. 2007.

55. Naghshineh N, Brown S, Cederna PS, et al. Demystifying the US Food and Drug Administration: understanding regulatory pathways. Plast Reconstr Surg 2014;134(3):559–69.

56. Schipper BM, Marra KG, Zhang W, et al. Regional anatomic and age effects on cell function of human adipose-derived stem cells. Ann Plast Surg 2008; 60(5):538–44.

57. Minteer DM, Gerlach JC, Marra KG. Bioreactors addressing diabetes mellitus. J Diabetes Sci Technol 2014;8(6):1227–32.

58. Patrick C, Uthamanthil R, Beahm E, et al. Animal models for adipose tissue engineering. Tissue Eng Part B Rev 2008;14:167–78.

59. Clavijo-Alvarez JA, Rubin JP, Bennett J, et al. A novel perfluoroelastomer seeded with adipose-derived stem cells for soft-tissue repair. Plast Reconstr Surg 2006;118:1132.

60. Thesleff T, Lehtimaki K, Niskakangas T, et al. Cranioplasty with adipose-derived stem cells and biomaterial: a novel method for cranial reconstruction. Neurosurgery 2011;68:1535–40.

61. Mesimaki K, Lindroos B, Tornwall J, et al. Novel maxillary reconstruction with ectopic bone formation by GMP adipose stem cells. Int J Oral Maxillofac Surg 2009;38:201–9.

62. Lee K, Kim H, Kim JM, et al. Systemic transplantation of human adipose-derived stem cells stimulates bone repair by promoting osteoblast and osteoclast function. J Cell Mol Med 2011;15: 2082–94.

63. Levi B, James AW, Nelson ER, et al. Acute skeletal injury is necessary for human adipose-derived stromal cell-mediated calvarial regeneration. Plast Reconstr Surg 2011;127:1118–29.

64. Levi B, James AW, Nelson ER, et al. Human adipose derived stromal cells heal critical size mouse calvarial defects. PLoS One 2010;5:E11177.

65. Cowan CM, Shi YY, Aalami OO, et al. Adipose-derived adult stromal cells heal critical-size mouse calvarial defects. Nat Biotechnol 2004; 22:560–7. Landmark study documenting the utility of ASCs for the repair of a murine cranial bone defects.

66. Lendeckel S, Jodicke A, Christophis P, et al. Autologous stem cells (adipose) and fibrin glue used to treat widespread traumatic calvarial defects: case report. J Craniomaxillofac Surg 2004;32:370–3.

67. Bai X, Alt E. Myocardial regeneration potential of adipose tissue-derived stem cells. Biochem Biophys Res Commun 2010;401:321–6.

68. Mazo M, Gavira JJ, Pelacho B, et al. Adipose-derived stem cells for myocardial infarction. J Cardiovasc Transl Res 2011;4:145–53.

69. Bai X, Yan Y, Song YH, et al. Both cultured and freshly isolated adipose tissue-derived stem cells enhance cardiac function after acute myocardial infarction. Eur Heart J 2010;31:489–501.

70. Bai X, Yan Y, Coleman M, et al. Tracking long-term survival of intramyocardially delivered human adipose tissue-derived stem cells using bioluminescence imaging. Mol Imaging Biol 2011;13:633–45.

71. Ii M, Horii M, Yokoyama A, et al. Synergistic effect of adipose-derived stem cell therapy and bone marrow progenitor recruitment in ischemic heart. Lab Invest 2010;91(4):539–52.

72. Bayes-Genis A, Soler-Botija C, Farre J, et al. Human progenitor cells derived from cardiac adipose tissue ameliorate myocardial infarction in rodents. J Mol Cell Cardiol 2010;49:771–80.

73. Gaebel R, Furlani D, Sorg H, et al. Cell origin of human mesenchymal stem cells determines a different healing performance in cardiac regeneration. PLoS One 2011;6:E15652.

74. Alt E, Pinkernell K, Scharlau M, et al. Effect of freshly isolated autologous tissue resident stromal cells on cardiac function and perfusion following acute myocardial infarction. Int J Cardiol 2010; 144:26–35.

75. Fotuhi P, Song YH, Alt E. Electrophysiological consequence of adipose-derived stem cell transplantation in infarcted porcine myocardium. Europace 2007;9:1218–21.

76. Valina C, Pinkernell K, Song YH, et al. Intracoronary administration of autologous adipose tissue-derived stem cells improves left ventricular function, perfusion, and remodelling after acute myocardial infarction. Eur Heart J 2007;28:2667–77.

77. Bel A, Planat-Bernard V, Saito A, et al. Composite cell sheets: a further step toward safe and effective myocardial regeneration by cardiac progenitors derived from embryonic stem cells. Circulation 2010;122:S118–23.

78. Eto H, Suga H, Inoue K, et al. Adipose injury-associated factors mitigate hypoxia in ischemic tissues through activation of adipose-derived stem/progenitor/stromal cells and induction of angiogenesis. Am J Pathol 2011;178:2322–32.

79. Yang YC, Liu BS, Shen CC, et al. Transplantation of adipose tissue-derived stem cells for treatment of focal cerebral ischemia. Curr Neurovasc Res 2011;8:1–13.

80. Lewis DS, Soderstrom PG. In vivo and in vitro development of visceral adipose tissue in a nonhuman primate (*Papio* species). Metabolism 1993;42:1277–83.

81. Zuk PA. Viral transduction of adipose-derived stem cells. Methods Mol Biol 2011;702:345–57.

82. Choi EW, Shin IS, Lee HW, et al. Transplantation of CTLA4Ig gene-transduced adipose tissue-derived mesenchymal stem cells reduces inflammatory immune response and improves Th1/Th2 balance in experimental autoimmune thyroiditis. J Gene Med 2011;13:3–16.

83. McIntosh K, Zvonic S, Garrett S, et al. The immunogenicity of human adipose derived cells: temporal changes in vitro. Stem Cells 2006;24:1245–53.

84. Puissant B, Barreau C, Bourin P, et al. Immunomodulatory effect of human adipose tissue-derived adult stem cells: comparison with bone marrow mesenchymal stem cells. Br J Haematol 2005;129:118–29.

85. Riordan NH, Ichim TE, Min WP, et al. Non-expanded adipose stromal vascular fraction cell therapy for multiple sclerosis. J Transl Med 2009;7:29.

86. Bartholomew A, Sturgeon C, Siatskas M, et al. Mesenchymal stem cells suppress lymphocyte proliferation in vitro and prolong skin graft survival in vivo. Exp Hematol 2002;30:42–8.

87. Ivanova-Todorova E, Bochev I, Mourdjeva M, et al. Adipose tissue-derived mesenchymal stem cells are more potent suppressors of dendritic cells differentiation compared with bone marrow-derived mesenchymal stem cells. Immunol Lett 2009;126:37–42.

88. DelaRosa O, Lombardo E, Beraza A, et al. Requirement of IFN-gamma-mediated indoleamine 2,3-dioxygenase expression in the modulation of lymphocyte proliferation by human adipose-derived stem cells. Tissue Eng Part A 2009;15:2795–806.

89. Shi D, Liao L, Zhang B, et al. Human adipose tissue-derived mesenchymal stem cells facilitate the immunosuppressive effect of cyclosporin A on T lymphocytes through Jagged-1-mediated inhibition of NF-κB signaling. Exp Hematol 2011;39:214–24.

90. Crop MJ, Baan CC, Korevaar SS, et al. Human adipose tissue-derived mesenchymal stem cells induce explosive T-cell proliferation. Stem Cells Dev 2010;19:1843–53.

91. Kronsteiner B, Wolbank S, Peterbauer A, et al. Human mesenchymal stem cells from adipose tissue and amnion influence T-cells depending on stimulation method and presence of other immune cells. Stem Cells Dev 2011;20(12):2115–26.

92. Technau A, Froelich K, Hagen R, et al. Adipose tissue-derived stem cells show both immunogenic and immunosuppressive properties after chondrogenic differentiation. Cytotherapy 2011;13:310–7.

93. Calderon D, Planat-Benard V, Bellamy V, et al. Immune response to human embryonic stem cell-derived cardiac progenitors and adipose-derived stromal cells. J Cell Mol Med 2011;16(7):1544–52.

94. Choi EW, Shin IS, Park SY, et al. Reversal of serological, immunological and histological dysfunction in systemic lupus erythematosus mice by long-term serial adipose tissue-derived mesenchymal stem cell transplantation. Arthritis Rheum 2012;64(1):243–53.

95. Gonzalez MA, Gonzalez-Rey E, Rico L, et al. Treatment of experimental arthritis by inducing immune tolerance with human adipose-derived mesenchymal stem cells. Arthritis Rheum 2009;60:1006–19.

96. Gonzalez-Rey E, Gonzalez MA, Varela N, et al. Human adipose-derived mesenchymal stem cells reduce inflammatory and T-cell responses and induce regulatory T cells in vitro in rheumatoid arthritis. Ann Rheum Dis 2010;69:241–8.

97. Gonzalez MA, Gonzalez-Rey E, Rico L, et al. Adipose-derived mesenchymal stem cells alleviate experimental colitis by inhibiting inflammatory and autoimmune responses. Gastroenterology 2009;136:978–89.

98. Gonzalez-Rey E, Anderson P, Gonzalez MA, et al. Human adult stem cells derived from adipose tissue protect against experimental colitis and sepsis. Gut 2009;58:929–39.

99. Garcia-Olmo D, Garcia-Arranz M, Garcia LG, et al. Autologous stem cell transplantation for treatment of rectovaginal fistula in perianal Crohn's disease: a new cell-based therapy. Int J Colorectal Dis 2003;18:451–4.

100. Garcia-Olmo D, Garcia-Arranz M, Herreros D. Expanded adipose-derived stem cells for the treatment of complex perianal fistula including Crohn's disease. Expert Opin Biol Ther 2008;8:1417–23.

101. Garcia-Olmo D, Garcia-Arranz M, Herreros D, et al. A Phase I clinical trial of the treatment of Crohn's fistula by adipose mesenchymal stem cell transplantation. Dis Colon Rectum 2005;48:1416–23.

102. Garcia-Olmo D, Herreros D, Pascual I, et al. Expanded adipose-derived stem cells for the treatment of complex perianal fistula: a phase II clinical trial. Dis Colon Rectum 2009;52:79–86.

103. Garcia-Olmo D, Herreros D, Pascual M, et al. Treatment of enterocutaneous fistula in Crohn's disease with adipose-derived stem cells: a comparison of protocols with and without cell expansion. Int J Colorectal Dis 2009;24:27–30.

104. Constantin G, Marconi S, Rossi B, et al. Adipose-derived mesenchymal stem cells ameliorate chronic experimental autoimmune encephalomyelitis. Stem Cells 2009;27:2624–35.

105. Kang HM, Kim J, Park S, et al. Insulin-secreting cells from human eyelid-derived stem cells alleviate type I diabetes in immunocompetent mice. Stem Cells 2009;27:1999–2008.

106. Chandra V, G S, Phadnis S, et al. Generation of pancreatic hormone-expressing islet-like cell aggregates from murine adipose tissue-derived stem cells. Stem Cells 2009;27:1941–53.

107. Chandra V, Swetha G, Muthyala S, et al. Islet-like cell aggregates generated from human adipose tissue derived stem cells ameliorate experimental diabetes in mice. PLoS One 2011;6:E20615.

108. Ohmura Y, Tanemura M, Kawaguchi N, et al. Combined transplantation of pancreatic islets and adipose tissue-derived stem cells enhances the survival and insulin function of islet grafts in diabetic mice. Transplantation 2010;90:1366–73.

109. Fumimoto Y, Matsuyama A, Komoda H, et al. Creation of a rich subcutaneous vascular network with implanted adipose tissue-derived stromal cells and adipose tissue enhances subcutaneous grafting of islets in diabetic mice. Tissue Eng Part C Methods 2009;15:437–44.

110. Fang B, Song Y, Liao L, et al. Favorable response to human adipose tissue-derived mesenchymal stem cells in steroid-refractory acute graft-versus-host disease. Transplant Proc 2007;39:3358–62.

111. NIH. Registry and results database of federally and privately supported clinical trials conducted in the United States. 2014. Available at: http://www.clinicaltrials.gov. Accessed December 15, 2014.

112. Meirelles Lda S, Fontes AM, Covas DT, et al. Mechanisms involved in the therapeutic properties of mesenchymal stem cells. Cytokine Growth Factor Rev 2009;20:419–27.

113. Gimble JM, Bunnell BA, Guilak F. Human adipose-derived cells: an update on the transition to clinical translation. Regen Med 2012;7(2):225–35.

114. Sensebe L, Bourin P. Producing MSC according GMP: process and controls. Biomed Mater Eng 2008;18:173–7.

115. Sensebe L, Bourin P, Tarte K. Good manufacturing practices production of mesenchymal stem/stromal cells. Hum Gene Ther 2011;22:19–26.

116. Bourin P, Gadelorge M, Peyrafitte JA, et al. Mesenchymal progenitor cells: tissue origin, isolation and culture. Transfus Med Hemother 2008;35:160–7.

117. Reed W, Noga SJ, Gee AP, et al. Production Assistance for Cellular Therapies (PACT): four-year experience from the United States National Heart, Lung, and Blood Institute (NHLBI) contract research program in cell and tissue therapies. Transfusion 2009;49(4):786–96.

How Does Fat Survive and Remodel After Grafting?

Takanobu Mashiko, MD, Kotaro Yoshimura, MD*

KEYWORDS

- Fat grafting • Adipose-derived stem/stromal cell • Tissue regeneration • Macrophages
- Vascular endothelial cells

KEY POINTS

- Under severe ischemia, adipocytes die within 24 hours; adipose-derived stem/stromal cells (ASCs) survive up to 3 days and are activated, contributing to the repairing process through adipogenesis, angiogenesis, and paracrine effects.
- Adipocyte fate after fat grafting is categorized into three zones depending on the distance from the surface: survival, regeneration, and necrosis.
- ASCs do not die and give rise to new adipocytes in the regenerating zone; they die in the necrotizing zone. The balance between regeneration and degeneration determines the final volume retention after fat grafting.
- Dead adipocytes under better conditions (regenerating zone) are phagocytized by macrophages and are successfully replaced by new adipocytes.
- Dead adipocytes under worse conditions (necrotizing zone) are replaced with cicatrization or oil cyst formation depending on the size of oil drops.

INTRODUCTION

Adipose tissue and adipose-derived stem/stromal cells (ASCs) obtained from liposuction were shown to have potential for regenerative therapeutic use. However, clinical outcomes of fat grafting remain unpredictable and, to improve the outcomes, it is crucial to elucidate the detailed mechanism of engraftment of fat tissue. The "cell survival theory," which maintains that transplanted adipocytes partly survive once they receive adequate nutrients and remain alive in the recipient site, had been accepted for a long time.[1-3] In contrast, our recent studies showed how ASCs work in response to microenvironmental changes, such as ischemia and applied mechanical force,[4,5] and revealed the "cell replacement theory," which holds that most adipocytes undergo ischemic death and subsequent replacement with next generation during the first 3 months after fat grafting.[6,7] Further details, such as the cellular origin of adipose regeneration and the mechanism of cicatrization and oil cyst formation, were also demonstrated.[7]

BASIC SCIENCE: FUNCTIONAL ROLES OF ADIPOSE-DERIVED STEM/STROMAL CELLS IN TISSUE REMODELING
Adipose Tissue Biology

Adipose tissue is not only an organ of energy storage, but also an endocrine organ (releasing multiple adipose-derived hormones, such as leptin and adiponectin) that regulates metabolic

Financial Disclosure: Authors report no commercial associations or financial disclosures with regard to this article.

Department of Plastic Surgery, School of Medicine, University of Tokyo, 7-3-1, Hongo, Bunkyo-Ku, Tokyo 113-8655, Japan

* Corresponding author.

E-mail address: kotaro-yoshimura@umin.ac.jp

plasticsurgery.theclinics.com

homeostasis. Adipose tissue consists predominantly of adipocytes, ASCs, vascular endothelial cells (VECs), pericytes, fibroblasts, and connective tissue as well as adipose tissue-resident macrophages and lymphocytes (**Fig. 1**).[8] Our rough estimation of cellular component numbers are as follows; 1 cm³ intact adipose tissue contains several millions cells; 1 million adipocytes, 1 million ASCs, 1 million VECs, and 1 million other cells (adipose-resident macrophages and lymphocytes, pericytes, fibroblasts, etc).[8] Adipose tissue is rich in capillary and every single adipocyte is attached to the capillary network. The size of adipocyte is 50 to 150 μm in diameter (if it becomes larger, it dies from ischemia) and its life span is several to 10 years in humans. ASCs are located perivascularly along the capillaries between adipocytes like pericytes. ASCs have been shown to release angiogenic factors responding to ischemia[4] and to differentiate physiologically into adipocytes and VECs.[9] A small subpopulation of ASCs (1%–2%) may have greater multipotency, corresponding with stem cells called multilineage differentiating stress enduring (Muse) cells.[10] The enlarged adipocytes in obese individuals occasionally die from relative ischemia and are subsequently surrounded by infiltrated M1 inflammatory macrophages (crownlike structure). The crownlike structure is seen after any types of adipocyte death (**Fig. 2**).

Adipose-Derived Stem/Progenitor Cells in Adipose Tissue Remodeling

ASCs are the main cell population contributing to adipocyte (re)generation in any types of adipose tissue remodeling/expansion, such as developmental growth, hyperplasia in obesity, repair processes after injury/ischemia,[4] or tissue expansion induced by internal/external mechanical forces.[5] These remodeling processes are in balance between adipocyte apoptosis/necrosis and adipogenesis managed by ASCs. In ASC-deficient tissues, such as irradiated or chronically inflamed tissues, any type of adipose tissue remodeling or expansion is impaired and thus fat grafting to fertilize such stem cell–depleted condition would be theoretically the right solution.[11] Adipose-tissue atrophy over aging is likely owing to a decrease in number of ASCs and consequent impaired physiologic turnover, as is commonly seen in other tissues and organs.

Ischemia to Adipose Tissue

Subcutaneous adipose tissue has the highest tissue partial oxygen tension (ptO_2; 40–60 mm Hg) among organs. The high ptO_2 of adipose tissue probably reflects high density of capillaries and low oxygen consumption rate of the tissue. Diabetic adipose tissue is relatively ischemic with low-grade chronic inflammation, which causes

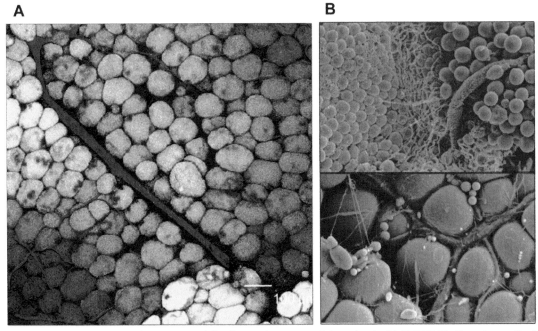

Fig. 1. Structure of human adipose tissue. (*A*) Adipose tissues are triple stained with BODIPY (adipocytes; *yellow*), lectin (endothelial cells; *red*), and Hoechst 33,342 (nuclei; *blue*). Adipose tissue is packed with adipocytes with scarce connective tissue and is rich in capillary network, though each adipocyte is exceptionally large in size. Scale bars = 100 μm. (*B*) Scanning electromicroscopic images.

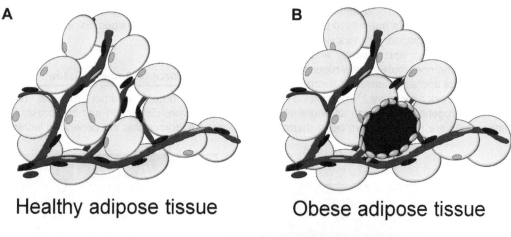

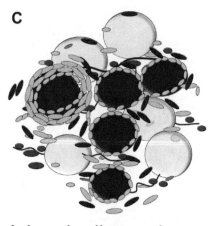

Injured adipose tissue

Fig. 2. Schema for structure of intact, obese, and injured adipose tissues. (*A*) Intact adipose tissue has not only adipocytes but also many other types of cells such as ASCs and vascular endothelial cells. (*B*) Obese adipose tissue has some dead adipocytes surrounded by infiltrated M1 macrophages (crownlike structure) and shows low-grade chronic inflammatory condition. (*C*) In injured adipose tissue, ASCs are activated and many types of progenitor/stem cells are recruited from bone marrow to repair the tissue damage. MSC, mesenchymal stem cell.

adipose endocrine dysfunction, insulin resistance, and the metabolic syndrome, whereas lipoma tissue is not ischemic, probably owing to upregulated angiogenesis.[12]

Among cellular components of adipose tissue, adipocytes are most susceptible to death under ischemic conditions such as 15 mm Hg of ptO_2.[6] When severe ischemia prolongs, VECs and blood-derived cells start to die next. In contrast, ASCs can remain alive up to 3 days, even under severely ischemic conditions.[6] Over the 3 days, they can be activated by signals from dying cells and contribute to the adaptive repairing process, such as by adipogenesis and angiogenesis.[6,7]

Injury to Adipose Tissue

Tissue injury also causes adipose tissue degeneration with inflammatory cell recruitment and release of inflammatory cytokines. After injury, degenerative changes such as adipocyte death occur, and primary injury factors such as basic fibroblast growth factor and other factors from aggregated platelets such as platelet-derived growth factor, epidermal growth factor, and transforming growth factor-β are first released into the injured site and trigger a cascade of wound healing processes.[4,13] Basic fibroblast growth factor is released from damaged connective tissue and acts through a c-Jun N-terminal kinase signaling pathway to stimulate ASCs not only to proliferate, but also to secrete secondary factors such as hepatocyte growth factor and vascular endothelial growth factor, and contributes to the regeneration of adipose tissue and suppression of fibrogenesis during the first week after injury.[13] In parallel, a variety of stem/progenitor cells such as endothelial progenitor cells are recruited from bone marrow and collaborate with activated ASCs in an orchestrated repair of the damaged adipose tissue (see **Fig. 2**).

Mechanical Force to Adipose Tissue

Mechanical forces, whether external (shear, stretch, tension, distraction and compression) or endogenous (forces that are generated within the

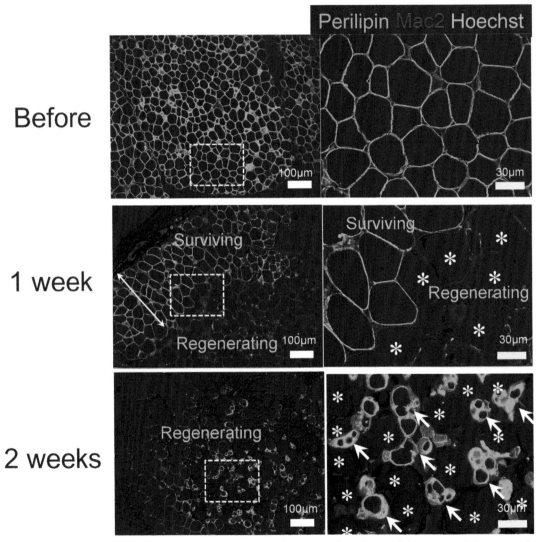

Fig. 3. Immunohistology of grafted fat tissue in mice (Before, 1 week and 2 weeks). Harvested tissue samples [before (*top*), 1 week (*middle*), and 2 weeks (*bottom*) after grafting] were immunostained for perilipin (cytoplasm of viable adipocytes; *green*), MAC2 (monocytes/macrophages; *red*) and Hoechst 33,342 (nuclei; *blue*). Rectangles in the low magnification images (*left column; yellow* scale bars = 100 μm) were further magnified in the right column (*white scale bars* = 30 μm). Demarcation between the surviving and regenerating zone became clear at 1 week (*interrupted line*); dead adipocytes (*asterisk*) were perilipin negative and surviving adipocytes were strongly positive for perilipin. Small-sized preadipocytes with multiple intracellular lipid droplets (*arrows*) appeared between dead adipocytes at 2 weeks; the dead adipocytes were surrounded by a single layer of macrophages (*red*). (*Adapted from* Kato H, Mineda K, Eto H, et al. Degeneration, regeneration, and cicatrization after fat grafting: dynamic total tissue remodeling during the first 3 months. Plast Reconstr Surg 2014;133:306e; with permission.)

active cytoskeleton), affect tissue growth, cellular function, and even survival. Moreover, physical interactions with the extracellular matrix can significantly influence stem cell behavior.[14] Continuous external tissue expansion (Brava®) is attempted for expansion of the breast tissue.[15] Experimentally, 4 weeks of external suspension caused enlargement of the subcutaneous tissue, particularly adipose tissue, although the enlargement was reversible.[5] The regenerating potential has been attributed to the number (density) and potential of ASCs; thus, irradiated tissue has a limited potential for expansion.

RELEVANCE TO CLINICIANS: WHAT HAPPENS AFTER FAT GRAFTING?
Acute Events Immediately After Fat Grafting

The grafted nonvascularized adipose tissue is placed under ischemia (hypoxia) and is nourished only by plasmatic diffusion from the surrounding host tissue for a few days until revascularization occurs. This results in the death of many adipocytes within 24 hours and release of multiple cell death and injury-associated factors from the dying donor tissue and injured host tissue (**Fig. 3**).[6,13] Inflammatory cells, such as macrophages and lymphocytes, are infiltrated and inflammatory cytokines, such as interleukins, are secreted. Despite the death of adipocytes, ASCs, which can be functional for up to 72 hours even under severe ischemia, are activated and try to repair the damaged tissue in collaboration with infiltrated stem and progenitor cells from the bone marrow.[6,7]

Regeneration After Ischemic Tissue Damage: Three Zones with Differential Cell Fates

Based on our recent studies, the first 3 months after fat grafting is a period of tissue remodeling; adipogenesis does not occur after this period.[11] The grafted fat is categorized into three zones from the periphery to the center: (1) survival (superficial), (2) regeneration (intermediate), and (3) necrosis (central; **Fig. 4**).[7] The demarcation of the surviving zone (100–300 μm thick) from the regenerating

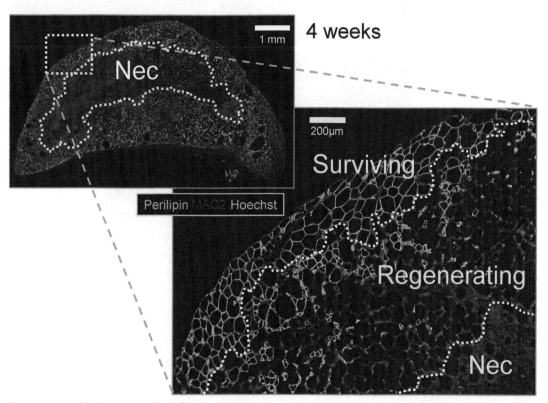

Fig. 4. Immunohistology of grafted fat tissue in mice (4 weeks). Immunohistology of a graft sample at 4 weeks showed demarcated surviving, regenerating, and necrotizing zones. (*Left, above*) A low-magnification image of perilipin staining showed the necrotizing zone (*yellow interrupted line*) with no adipogenesis. White scale bar = 1 mm. (*Right, below*) A high-magnification image showed demarcated (with *white interrupted lines*) surviving (perilipin-positive adipocytes), regenerating (perilipin-positive small adipocytes), and necrotizing zones (no viable adipocytes). Yellow scale bar = 100 μm.

zone became clear at 1 week, whereas the demarcation between the regenerating and necrotizing zones was obvious between 2 and 4 weeks (see **Fig. 3**).

Adipocytes superficially located 100 to 300 μm from the tissue edge remain alive (surviving zone), and all the rest of adipocytes (regenerating and necrotizing zones) die within 24 hours after grafting. The dead adipocytes are surrounded by M1 macrophages for phagocytosis (see **Fig. 3**), but the absorption process takes weeks or months, depending on the size and therefore the grafted fat maintains its original size for the first 4 weeks despite adipocyte death. ASCs in the regenerating and necrotizing zones are activated and start to repair the tissue. New, small preadipocytes appeared around the dead adipocytes (surrounded by a single layer of macrophages) at 1 to 2 weeks in the regenerating zone (600–1200 μm thick),

whereas no adipogenesis was observed in the necrotizing zone (see **Fig. 4**). In the regenerating zone, the hypoxic condition is improved by revascularization within 3 days and ASCs give rise to new adipocytes, which finally replace the dead adipocytes by 3 months. On the other hand, in the necrotizing zone, the microenvironment is not improved within 3 days and ASCs also die, leading to central necrosis of the graft tissue.

The ratio between the necrotizing and surviving/regenerating zones, which determines the final volume retention after fat grafting, varies depending on the recipient microenvironment, based on factors such as vascularity, as well as the size of the grafted fat, grafting technique, and postoperative care. Our experimental study using a mouse model revealed that oxygenation of the recipient bed with normobaric 60% oxygen for 3 days postoperatively promotes survival, regeneration, and

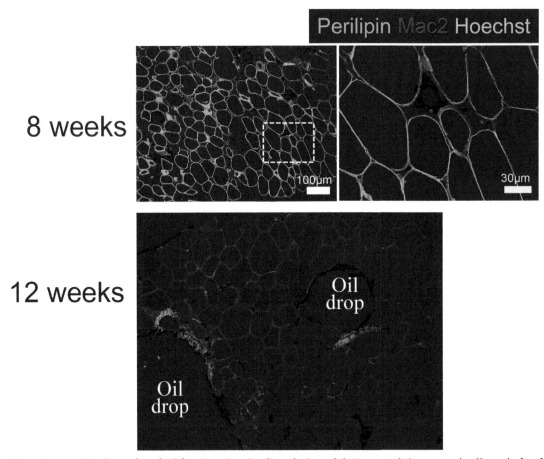

Fig. 5. Immunohistology of grafted fat tissue in mice (8 and 12 weeks). Harvested tissue samples (8 weeks [*top*] and 12 weeks [*bottom*] after grafting) were immunostained for perilipin (cytoplasm of viable adipocytes; *green*), MAC2 (monocytes/macrophages; *red*) and Hoechst 33,342 (nuclei; *blue*). There are few small new adipocytes, which means that adipose regeneration seemed to be finished by 12 weeks. Large-sized lipid drops surrounded by M1 macrophages are left in the tissue. (*Modified from* Kato H, Mineda K, Eto H, et al. Degeneration, regeneration, and cicatrization after fat grafting: dynamic total tissue remodeling during the first 3 months. Plast Reconstr Surg 2014;133:306e.)

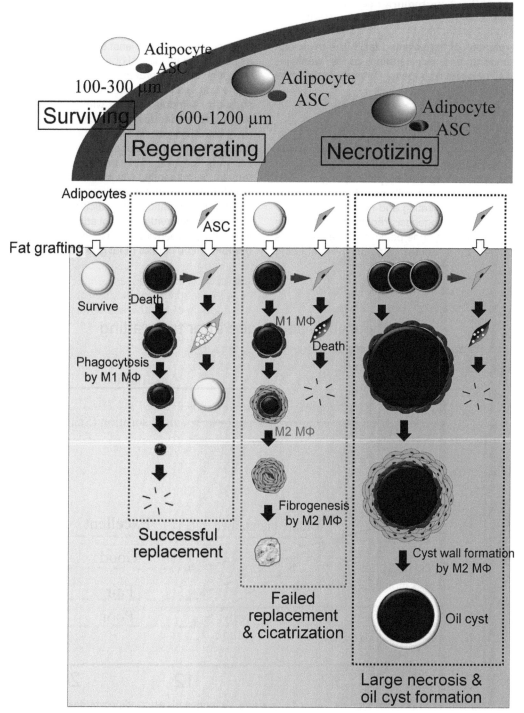

Fig. 6. Conclusive schema for the fate of adipocytes in grafted fat. During the first 3 months of adipose tissue remodeling, transplanted adipocytes have differential fates depending on their microenvironments. In this schema, complex cellular events are simplified and the adipocyte fate is categorized into 4 patterns: survival, successful regeneration, failed regeneration (cicatrization), and oil cyst formation. Cicatrization and oil cyst formation are often not complete at 3 months. The most superficial zone is the "surviving zone," which is less than 300 μm thick. In the surviving zone, both adipocytes and adipose-derived stem cells (ASCs) survive. The second zone is the "regenerating zone," the thickness of which varies (600–1200 μm) depending on the microenvironmental conditions. In this zone, adipocytes die, but ASCs survive and provide new adipocytes to replace the dead ones. The most central zone is the "necrosis zone," where both adipocytes and ASCs die, no regeneration is expected, and the dead space will be absorbed, be filled with fibrosis, or develop into an oil cyst. (*Modified from* Kato H, Mineda K, Eto H, et al. Degeneration, regeneration, and cicatrization after fat grafting: dynamic total tissue remodeling during the first 3 months. Plast Reconstr Surg 2014;133:312e.)

final retention of transplanted fat.[16] The thickness of surviving and regenerating zones were increased, suggesting superior survival of adipocyte and resident ASCs, respectively.

Long-Term Stabilization Process (Lipid Absorption and Cicatrization)

In parallel with the regenerating events, stabilizing events, such as lipid absorption (phagocytosis) and lipid replacement with scar tissue (fibrosis), occur in the regenerating and necrotizing zones.[7] Although the adipogenesis/regeneration process in the regenerating zone peaks at 4 weeks and is completed by 3 months (**Fig. 5**), the stabilizing process persists for at least several more months, as suggested by clinical observations that volume reduction after fat grafting continues until the end of the first year. Small-sized oil droplets were absorbed or temporarily filled with multilayered M2 macrophages, inducing the dead space replacement with fibrogenesis in parallel with lipid absorption. On the contrary, substantially larger oil drops (>8 mm) form oil cysts in several months and remain permanently, which are considered the worst outcome of fat grafting accompanied by chronic inflammation and calcification.[7,11,17] We summarize differential fates of adipocytes depending on the microenvironment in **Fig. 6** and the postoperative time course of fat grafting in **Fig. 7**.

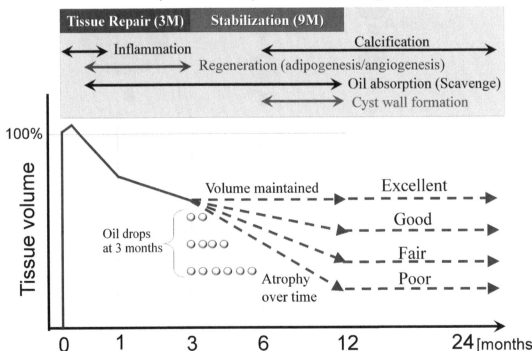

Fig. 7. Long-term postoperative sequence after fat grafting. Adipogenesis after adipocyte death is exerted by activated adipose-derived stem cells (ASCs). Some of the dead adipocytes are replaced with new adipocytes of next generation and the adipogenesis is finish by 3 months (tissue "repair" phase). Dead adipocytes remaining at 3 months are absorbed during the next 9 months (tissue "stabilization" phase). Lipid droplets (dead adipocytes) are absorbed by macrophage phagocytosis, but the absorption is very slow and the absorption period depends on the diameter of the lipid droplets; when the lipid droplet diameter was large, such as 10 mm, the cyst wall is formed before completing absorption and the cyst wall start to calcify over time. The final volume retention after fat grafting is determined by the rate of successful replacement of adipocytes. If grafted adipose has only small lipid droplets and absorption is finished by 3 months, the volume will not substantially change after 3 months (shown as "excellent"). On the other hand, many large lipid droplets remain at 3 months, tissue will atrophy between 3 and 12 months (shown as "poor"). (*Adapted from* Yoshimura K, Eto H, Kato H, et al. In vivo manipulation of stem cells for adipose tissue repair/reconstruction. Regen Med 2011;6(6 Suppl):38; with permission.)

What Are the Origins of Next-Generation Cells After Fat Grafting?

Our recent study using green fluorescent protein mice revealed the origin of cell components in grafted fat.[18] Mature adipocytes are mostly derived from ASCs in the graft. Although vascular wall constituents (smooth muscle cells) are chiefly graft derived; capillaries (VECs) originated equally from the graft and the host bone marrow. ASCs of the regenerated fat are an admixture of grafted, host non–bone marrow, and host bone marrow cells. These findings highlight the importance of ASCs contained in the grafted fat for regeneration of adipocytes. Also, host bone marrow and local tissues contribute substantially to capillary networks and the provision of new ASCs, which can contribute to future remodeling. Thus, although ASCs can be provided by bone marrow or other tissues, they have to get ready by staying adjacent to adipocytes in of contributing to adipocyte regeneration after adipocyte death.

Clinical Implications: How We Can Improve the Engraftment of Grafted Fat?

Recent advancements in the understanding of the underlying mechanisms provide a number of clinical implications. It is considered that the size and thickness of surviving zone are influenced by the surrounding recipient tissue. Better vascularity and greater oxygen tension of recipient tissue increase the surviving zone. Preconditioning of recipient tissue, negative pressure, and/or hyperoxygenation may help for this purpose. Excessively high internal pressure keeps the recipient tissue ischemic and reduces the surviving zone. As with skin grafts, immobilization should help the capillary to grow into the graft during the first week, which improves the oxygen tension of the regenerating zone and rescues ASCs from ischemic death. The size and surface area of grafted fat is a critical factor to minimize the central necrotizing zone; the diameter of grafted fat particles or noodles would be recommended to be as small as 2 mm. For adipogenesis after fat grafting, it is very important to have a good number of both viable adipocytes and ASCs in the graft (not helped from the outside). Adipocytes can release crucial factors to activate adjacent ASCs and lead them to differentiation into adipocytes. This finding strongly suggests that it is worth considering preparing a better number and ratio of adipocytes and ASCs during the tissue processing before grafting (discussed in the article by Kuno and Yoshimura elsewhere in this issue).

SUMMARY

ASCs act as main players in any types of adipose tissue regeneration, including after fat grafting, by differentiating into adipocytes or VECs and releasing angiogenic growth factors. The fate of grafted fat depends on its size and the microenvironment of cellular components, such as adipocytes. Adipocytes remain alive in the surviving zone, whereas they die shortly after grafting in the regenerating and necrotizing zones. Adjacent perivascular ASCs are activated by adipocyte death and begin to proliferate and differentiate to repair the damaged tissue in collaboration with infiltrated stem/progenitor cells in the regenerating zone. Dead adipocytes are phagocytized by M1 macrophages and are replaced successfully by new adipocytes without residual fibrosis in a better condition of the regenerating zone. In contrast, dead adipocytes under worse conditions in the regenerating or necrotizing zones are replaced partly with fibrosis or oil cysts; M2 macrophages act in the fibrogenesis process. Interestingly, dead adipocytes work as spacers and keep the space for new adipocytes during the regeneration process. The final volume retention after fat grafting is determined by the balance between degeneration and regeneration of adipose tissue and affected by many surgeons' factors including the microenvironments of graft regenerating zone and surrounding recipient tissue. Adipogenesis after fat grafting depends greatly on ASCs resident in the graft tissue, suggesting the importance of tissue processing before transplantation.

REFERENCES

1. Smahel J. Adipose tissue in plastic surgery. Ann Plast Surg 1986;16:444–53.
2. Billings E Jr, May JW Jr. Historical review and present status of free graft autotransplantation in plastic and reconstructive surgery. Plast Reconstr Surg 1989;83:368–81.
3. Cortese A, Savastano G, Felicetta L. Free fat transplantation for facial tissue augmentation. J Oral Maxillofac Surg 2000;58:164–9.
4. Suga H, Eto H, Shigeura T, et al. IFATS collection: fibroblast growth factor-2 induced hepatocyte growth factor secretion by adipose-derived stromal cells inhibits postinjury fibrogenesis through a c-Jun N-terminal kinase-dependent mechanism. Stem Cells 2009;27:238–49.
5. Kato H, Suga H, Eto H, et al. Reversible adipose tissue enlargement induced by external tissue suspension: possible contribution of basic fibroblast growth factor in the preservation of enlarged tissue. Tissue Eng Part A 2010;16:2029–40.

6. Eto H, Kato H, Suga H, et al. The fate of adipocytes after nonvascularized fat grafting: evidence of early death and replacement of adipocytes. Plast Reconstr Surg 2012;129:1081–92.

7. Kato H, Mineda K, Eto H, et al. Degeneration, regeneration, and cicatrization after fat grafting: dynamic total tissue remodeling during the first 3 months. Plast Reconstr Surg 2014;133:e303–13.

8. Eto H, Suga H, Matsumoto D, et al. Characterization of structure and cellular components of aspirated and excised adipose tissue. Plast Reconstr Surg 2009;124:1087–97.

9. Planat-Benard V, Silvestre JS, Cousin B, et al. Plasticity of human adipose lineage cells toward endothelial cells: physiological and therapeutic perspectives. Circulation 2004;109:656–63.

10. Ogura F, Wakao S, Kuroda Y, et al. Human adipose tissue possesses a unique population of pluripotent stem cells with nontumorigenic and low telomerase activities: potential implications in regenerative medicine. Stem Cells Dev 2014;23:717–28.

11. Yoshimura K, Eto H, Kato H, et al. In vivo manipulation of stem cells for adipose tissue repair/reconstruction. Regen Med 2011;6(6 Suppl):33–41.

12. Suga H, Eto H, Inoue K, et al. Cellular and molecular features of lipoma tissue: comparison with normal adipose tissue. Br J Dermatol 2009;161:819–25.

13. Eto H, Suga H, Aoi N, et al. Adipose injury-associated factors activate adipose stem/stromal cells, induce neoangiogenesis, and mitigate hypoxia in ischemic tissues. Am J Pathol 2011;178:2322–32.

14. Guilak F, Cohen DM, Estes BT, et al. Control of stem cell fate by physical interactions with the extracellular matrix. Cell Stem Cell 2009;5:17–26.

15. Khouri RK, Schlenz I, Murphy BJ, et al. Nonsurgical breast enlargement using an external soft-tissue expansion system. Plast Reconstr Surg 2000;105:2500–12.

16. Kato H, Araki J, Doi K, et al. Normobaric hyperoxygenation enhances initial survival, regeneration, and final retention in fat grafting. Plast Reconstr Surg 2014;134:951–9.

17. Mineda K, Kuno S, Kato H, et al. Chronic inflammation and progressive calcification as a result of fat necrosis: the worst outcome in fat grafting. Plast Reconstr Surg 2014;133:1064–72.

18. Doi K, Ogata F, Eto H, et al. Differential contributions of graft- and host-derived cells in tissue regeneration/remodeling after fat grafting. Plast Reconstr Surg, in press.

Condensation of Tissue and Stem Cells for Fat Grafting

Shinichiro Kuno, MD, Kotaro Yoshimura, MD*

KEYWORDS

- Fat grafting • Cell assisted lipotransfer • Adipose-derived stem/stromal cell • Tissue regeneration
- Macrophages • Vascular endothelial cells

KEY POINTS

- Adequate centrifugation purifies and condenses aspirated adipose tissue and improves graft retention.
- We can condense tissue by removing unnecessary components of grafted tissue through decantation, filtrations or centrifugation.
- Condensation of adipose-derived stem/stromal cells (ASCs) is important to get better adipocyte regeneration after fat grafting and achieve tissue revitalizing effects.
- ASCs can be condensed by reducing adipocytes from the graft through mechanical processing or strong centrifugation.
- Supplementation of stromal vascular fraction or ASCs can also improve ASC/adipocyte ratio in the graft and is expected to obtain better outcomes for tissue volumization and revitalization.

INTRODUCTION

Adipose tissue has many types of cells other than adipocytes, which can be extracted as a cell pellet called stromal vascular fraction (SVF) through collagenase digestion of aspirated adipose tissue. SVF contains adipose-derived stem/stromal cells (ASCs), vascular endothelial cells, pericytes, adipose-resident macrophages, lymphocytes, and so on.[1] ASCs are regarded as a potent tool for cell base therapies because they have biological functions such as multidirection differentiation, growth factor secretion, and immunomodulation, and can be obtained readily in a large amount through liposuction.

Condensation of grafting adipose tissue is a key to achieve better volumizing effects (better volume retention) by fat grafting. It is particularly important when these is a limitation of injection volume (eg, breast) owing to the limited skin envelop, because an injection of excessive volume leads to severe ischemia and fat necrosis. Condensation of grafting fat can be achieved by means of removal of unnecessary components, such as water, oil, dead cells, and blood cells. Because aspirated fat tissue is relatively poor in stem cells (ASCs),[2] condensation of ASCs in the graft is another issue for seeking better volumizing effects.

Recently, regenerative effects of fat grafting are appreciated by many clinicians. Stem cell–depleted tissues such as irradiated tissue, chronically inflammatory tissue, and ischemic fibrous tissue are improved by fat grafting in quality, vascularity, and healing and expanding capacity.[3,4] It has been reported frequently that hypertrophic scarring and

Financial Disclosure: Authors report no commercial associations or financial disclosures with regard to this article.
Department of Plastic Surgery, School of Medicine, University of Tokyo, 7-3-1, Hongo, Bunkyo-Ku, Tokyo 113-8655, Japan
* Corresponding author.
E-mail address: kotaro-yoshimura@umin.ac.jp

plasticsurgery.theclinics.com

scar contracture are softer and that skin hyper-pigmentation disappears after fat grafting.[5] Such regenerative/revitalizing effects of fat grafting are considered to be derived from ASCs in the tissue. Therefore, condensation of ASCs in the graft may be also crucial for such regenerating/revitalizing applications.

BASIC SCIENCE
Difference Between Aspirated Fat Tissue and Intact Adipose Tissue

Adipose tissue contains various types of cells including adipocytes and ASCs, as well as connective tissue (see the article by Mashiko and Yoshimura elsewhere in this issue for details). When surgeons aspirate fat, only fragile parts of adipose tissue are harvested through a suction cannula, whereas the honeycomb-like fibrous structures remain intact in the donor site.[6] The fibrous structure is predominantly composed of connective tissues and large vasculatures, which are considered to contain many ASCs. We have found that aspirated fat tissue contains only one-half the number of ASCs compared with intact fat tissue.[2] Stage-specific embryonic antigen-3–positive cells, which may be highly multipotent stem cells (muse cells),[7] locate around large vasculatures. These cells are also deficient in aspirated adipose tissue (unpublished data, Doi K et al, 2012). The relative deficiency of ASCs in aspirated fat tissue may be owing to (1) a substantial portion of ASCs being left in the donor tissue and (2) some ASCs being released into the fluid portion of liposuction aspirates, possibly owing to the act of an endogenous enzyme.[1,6] Thus, aspirated fat tissue is regarded as relatively ASC poor compared with intact fat tissue. This low ASC/adipocyte ratio may be a reason for long-term atrophy after fat grafting.[2]

Importance of Adipose-Derived Stem/Stromal Cells in the Grafted Tissue for Adipose Regeneration after Fat Grafting

ASCs have the potential to modulate or suppress immunoreaction,[8] differentiate into adipocytes,[9,10] vascular endothelial cells, or others and release angiogenic growth factors, such as hepatocyte growth factor and vascular endothelial growth factor, especially under hypoxic conditions.[11] ASCs were reported to contribute to angiogenesis during the adipose remodeling process after ischemia or fat grafting.[9–11] Our recent study using green fluorescent protein mice revealed that regenerated adipocytes after fat grafting are mostly originated from ASCs in the graft tissue, but not from other host-derived stem/progenitor cells, although new ASCs can be provided partly by bone marrow or

other tissues.[12] It was suggested that only ASCs originally located adjacent to dying adipocytes can become adipocytes, although other ASCs can contribute in other ways, such as angiogenesis or release of growth factors.

RELEVANCE TO CLINICIANS
Graft Tissue Condensation

Liposuction aspirates contain some components unnecessary for adipose tissue engraftment/regeneration; water, oil (broken adipocytes), and blood cells (red blood cells and white blood cells). It is recommended to remove such components and reduce the graft volume without reducing the number of viable adipocytes and ASCs; this is called condensation of graft tissue. Tissue condensation is important, especially when there is a maximum limit in graft volume, such as with breast augmentation. There are 3 major methods for graft tissue condensation: decantation (gravity sedimentation), filtration with or without a vacuum, and centrifugation. Among the 3, centrifugation is most effective to remove the water content without losing ASCs, although some adipocytes can be broken by the mechanical force and the resulting condensed fat may become more viscous and need higher pressure to inject through a small cannula (**Fig. 1**).[13] Oil released from damaged adipocytes causes inflammation-like foreign materials, suggesting that removal of oil should be important for better healing after fat grafting.

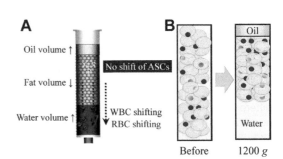

Fig. 1. Tissue and adipose-derived stem/stromal cell (ASC) condensation by centrifugation. (*A*) By centrifugation, fat volume becomes compact, water volume increases and oil will be clearly separated as a top layer. Many of red blood cells (RBCs) and white blood cells (WBCs) in the aspirated fat shift into the water portion after centrifugation, but most of ASCs remain in the fat portion. (*B*) By centrifugation at 1200×g for 3 minutes, fat volume decreases by 30%. Some adipocytes are broken and become oil as a top layer, but all ASCs remain intact and are concentrated in the condensed fat tissue.

Ratio of Adipocytes and Adipose-Derived Stem/Stromal Cells in the Graft

Recent studies indicate that ASCs in the graft are key components to contribute adipogenesis and angiogenesis after fat grafting. If the graft tissue is ASC deficient in number, it may be reasonable to normalize stem cell density in graft tissue.[6] There are theoretically 2 ways to improve the adipocyte/ASC ratio in the graft (ASC condensation): one is to reduce the number of adipocytes and tissue volume, and the other is to increase the number of ASCs (**Fig. 2**).

Reducing the number of adipocytes and tissue volume can be done by mechanical removal of adipocytes, such as mechanical crushing/mincing, aggressive centrifugation, and ultrasonic cavitation. Such destructive processes have to be done with great care, because too much damage, heat, or pressure to the tissue could kill ASCs as well. Increasing the number of ASCs can be done by supplementing freshly isolated SVF or cultured/purified ASCs to the graft (cell-assisted lipotransfer).[2] SVF can be achieved through collagenase digestion or other ways if extra liposuction aspirates are available. ASCs can be purified readily and expanded by adherent culture of SVF, and can also be banked in a liquid nitrogen for a long period if needed.

Adipose-Derived Stem/Stromal Cells Condensation by Reduction of Adipocytes and Tissue Volume

Reduction of adipocyte number in the tissue without losing ASC viability, which leads to tissue volume reduction and ASC condensation at the same time, can be done by various methods, such as aggressive centrifugation, mechanical crushing or mincing, and ultrasound cavitation.

Centrifugation not only separates water and oil from fat tissue, but also mechanically breaks some adipocytes, depending on the magnitude of centrifugal force, although ASCs in the tissue

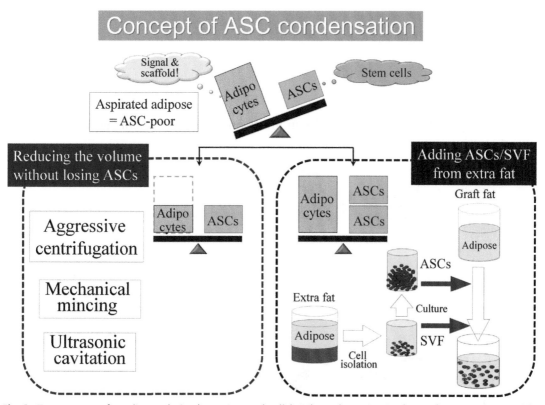

Fig. 2. Two concepts for adipose-derived stem/stromal cell (ASC) condensation in the graft tissue. Aspirated fat tissue is relatively ASC-poor compared with intact adipose tissue, and there are 2 concepts to normalize the ASC number in the tissue. One is to reduce the number of adipocytes without losing ASCs, which results in substantial volume reduction. After this process, adipose tissue and ASCs are condensed with a greater ratio of ASCs/adipocytes. Another is to supplement freshly isolated stromal vascular fraction (SVF) or culture expanded ASCs. Isolated ASCs cannot function unless they are properly incorporated into the tissue.

are well preserved when centrifuged at below 3000×g.[13] Thus, the adipocyte/ASC ratio can be increased after strong centrifugation (by 20% when centrifuged at 1200×g; see **Fig. 1**B). Adequate centrifugation condenses tissue and ASCs, and also improves fat graft survival, although too strong centrifugation may worsen graft survival.[13,14]

There are some other attempts to further condense adipose graft tissue. Mechanical chopping, shredding, pureeing, or mincing, manually or with specific devices (like homogenizers or food processors), can further fragment aspirated fat tissue and rupture adipocytes. Appropriately, such mechanical processing can reduce substantially adipocytes, which become oil and can be removed by subsequent centrifugation. As a result, condensed fat tissue with a reduced volume can be obtained, although excessive processing can kill ASCs as well as endothelial cells, and has to be avoided. Ultrasonic cavitation may be also useful to damage selectively adipocytes in the future.

Adipose-Derived Stem/Stromal Cells Condensation by Supplementing Stromal Vascular Fraction or Adipose-Derived Stem/Stromal Cells

Another strategy is supplementing freshly isolated SVF or culture-expanded ASCs to aspirated fat tissue and called cell-assisted (enhanced) lipotransfer (**Fig. 3**). We can achieve SVF cells from lipoaspirates through collagenase digestion (processed lipoaspirate cells), although a much smaller number of SVF is also obtained from the fluid infranatant portion of liposuction aspirates (liposuction aspirate fluid cells).[1] Other nonenzymatic methods, such as mechanical processing and ultrasonic cavitation, have been attempted, but there are no established, efficient methods so far.

Stromal Vascular Fraction Isolation Procedures

For processed lipoaspirate cells, suctioned fat tissue is digested with 0.075% collagenase in phosphate-buffered saline for 30 minutes on a

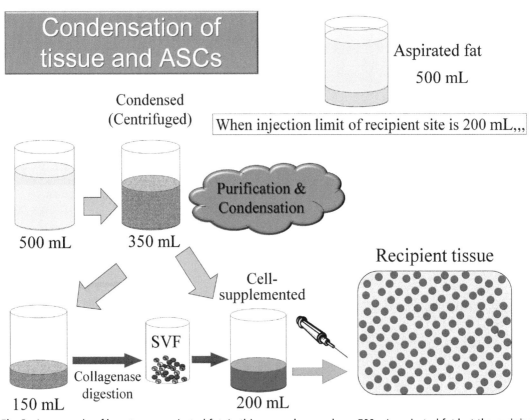

Fig. 3. An example of how to use aspirated fat. In this case, when we have 500 mL aspirated fat but the recipient tissue accepts a 200-mL injection at maximum (eg, owing to limited skin envelop), we can process and condense the graft tissue and adipose-derived stem/stromal cells (ASCs) before transplantation. Even after strong centrifugation, 350 mL of condensed fat tissue remains. Then the excessive 150 mL of centrifuged fat can be used for stromal vascular fraction (SVF) isolation for further condensation of ASCs in the graft material.

shaker at 37°C.[15] After centrifugation (800×g for 10 minutes), floating tissue (adipocytes and connective tissues) are discarded. The cell pellets are resuspended in Dulbecco's modified Eagle's medium and passed through a 100-mm mesh filter. To eliminate the remaining collagenase, the cells pellets are washed by resuspension in Dulbecco's modified Eagle's medium and after centrifugation at least 3 times. The process takes about 80 minutes (**Fig. 4**). For liposuction aspirate fluid cells, the suctioned fluid is centrifuged (400×g for 10 minutes) and the pellets are resuspended in distilled water (for 30 seconds) for erythrocyte lysis, followed by osmic normalization by adding 10% volume of 10× phosphate-buffered saline (or 9% NaCl solution). After centrifugation (and filtration), cell pellets are obtained as liposuction aspirate fluid cells; the process takes about 20 minutes. For these SVF cells, cell counting for erythrocytes and nucleated cells is performed using a hematocytometer used for blood testing. The SVF cell number is affected largely by hemorrhage contamination. Normal viable nucleate processed lipoaspirate cells cell number is 300,000 to 800,000 per 1 mL of aspirated adipose tissue.[1] Before injection, freshly isolated SVF cells or cultured ASCs are added to graft materials, followed by gentle mixing and a 5- to 10-minute incubation period to achieve appropriate cell adhesion to the graft tissue.

Clinical Reports of Cell-Assisted Lipotransfer

There are some studies reporting the clinical outcomes of cell-assisted lipotransfer. Although lipotransfer supplemented with ASCs or SVF cells have shown therapeutic potential in uncontrolled trials and comparative case series,[16–22] the clinical results remain controversial. Recently, some comparative studies of cell-assisted lipotransfer were reported. Chang and colleagues[23] reported a volumetric analysis of SVF-supplemented fat grafting and regular fat grafting to progressive hemifacial atrophy patients, concluding that fat survival and clinical improvement was greater with SVF-supplemented grafting than fat grafting alone after 6 months. Tanikawa and colleagues[24] reported that SVF-supplemented fat grafting for patients with craniofacial microsomia was effective. Survival fat volume was 88% at 6 months, which was significantly greater that nonsupplemented fat grafting (54%). Gentile and colleagues[25] applied SVF-supplemented fat grafting to the face and reported significantly better contouring maintenance compared with fat grafting alone. In contrast, Peltoniemi and colleagues[26] and Wang

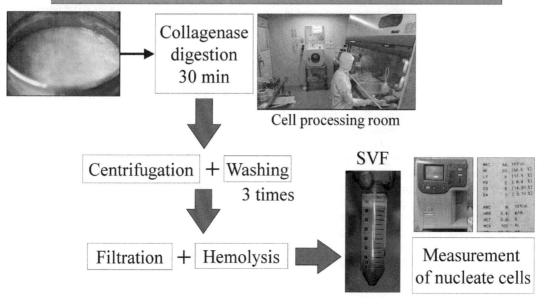

Fig. 4. Collagenase digestion process of aspirated fat for stromal vascular fraction (SVF) isolation. Aspirated fat is digested with collagenase for 30 minutes and the isolated cell fraction can be collected after spinning. Then, we wash the SVF cells, remove red blood cells by incubation with hemolysis buffer, and count the obtained nucleate cells with a hematocytometer or cell counter. The whole process should be performed in a clean room and takes about 80 minutes.

and colleagues[27] reported that cell-assisted lipo-transfer using SVF cells did not contribute to improve the outcomes.

Kølle and colleagues[28] reported a randomized, placebo-controlled trial to compare the volumizing effects of ASC-enhanced fat graft and regular fat graft in the same patients. In this study, ASCs were expanded by adherent culture and 20 million cultured ASCs were supplemented to 1 g fat graft, showing a significantly greater volume retention (80.9%) in ASC-supplemented group compared with 16.3% in the nonadditive control.

Taken together, the results of fat grafting with SVF/ASC supplementation seem to be affected by many factors. There is no standard or optimized method of SVF isolation and cell supplementation to the graft tissue. SVF contains many other cells, such as leukocytes, and some may have unfavorable effects on fat grafting. The number of ASCs isolated in SVF through collagenase is only 10% to 20% of those contained in the original tissue. ASCs have to be attached to the tissue or cells to function properly and avoid unwanted migration or differentiation.[29] Volume retention is not a reliable index to evaluate fat grafting results because oil cyst formation from large fat necrosis also increases the clinical score of volume retention. Further studies are necessary to achieve clinical benefits of ASCs with greater magnitude and consistency.

Further Condensation of Adipose-Derived Stem/Stromal Cells for Other Therapeutic Use

Fresh SVF and cultured ASCs have been used in numerous clinical trials, including autoimmune diseases, osteoarthritis, and myocardial infarction. These trials are expecting ASCs to reduce immunoreaction, release growth factors, and/or accelerate tissue repair and angiogenesis. However, there are other attempts to prepare ASC-containing tissues by removing adipocytes from adipose tissue and further condensing ASCs. Both adipocytes and ASCs are needed for tissue enlargement (adipose regeneration after fat grafting), but therapies for improving the quality (vascularity, inflammation, elasticity, and healing capacity) of tissue may not need any adipocytes. Fat grafting is showing clinical success for rejuvenating and revitalizing tissue. Such new types of processed adipose tissue (without adipocytes) are expected to be used in the future as an alternative to fat grafting for treating stem cell-depleted tissues.

SUMMARY

Adipose tissue has many types of cells other than adipocytes, which can be extracted as a cell pellet called SVF, which contains ASCs, vascular endothelial cells, pericytes, adipose-resident macrophages, and lymphocytes, among others. Condensation of grafting adipose tissue is a key to achieve better volumizing effects (better volume retention) by fat grafting. Because aspirated fat tissue is relatively poor in stem cells (ASCs), condensation of ASCs in the graft is another issue for seeking better volumizing and regenerating effects. One way to improve the adipocyte/ASC ratio in the graft (ASC condensation) is to reduce the number of adipocytes and tissue volume, and the other way is to increase the number of ASCs. ASC condensation can be done by mechanical removal of adipocytes, and increasing the number of ASCs can be achieved by supplementing freshly isolated SVF or cultured/purified ASCs to the graft (cell-assisted lipotransfer). Clinical trials of fat grafting with supplementation of SVF/ASCs suggested beneficial effects of supplementation, although further studies are needed to confirm and achieve benefits of ASCs with greater magnitude and consistency. For nonvolumizing purposes, such as revitalization of stem cell-depleted tissue and treatment of inflammatory conditions, a new style of processing of adipose tissue may be utilized in the future.

REFERENCES

1. Yoshimura K, Shigeura T, Matsumoto D, et al. Characterization of freshly isolated and cultured cells derived from the fatty and fluid portions of liposuction aspirates. J Cell Physiol 2006;208:64–76.
2. Matsumoto D, Sato K, Gonda K, et al. Cell-assisted lipotransfer: supportive use of human adipose-derived cells for soft tissue augmentation with lipoinjection. Tissue Eng 2006;12:3375–82.
3. Rigotti G, Marchi A, Galiè M, et al. Clinical treatment of radiotherapy tissue damage by lipoaspirate transplant: a healing process mediated by adipose-derived adult stem cells. Plast Reconstr Surg 2007;119:1409–22.
4. Salgarello M, Visconti G, Barone-Adesi L. Fat grafting and breast reconstruction with implant: another option for irradiated breast cancer patients. Plast Reconstr Surg 2012;129:317–29.
5. Caviggioli F, Maione L, Forcellini D, et al. Autologous fat graft in postmastectomy pain syndrome. Plast Reconstr Surg 2011;128:349–52.
6. Yoshimura K, Suga H, Eto H. Adipose-derived stem/progenitor cells: roles in adipose tissue remodeling and potential use for soft tissue augmentation. Regen Med 2009;4:265–73.
7. Kuroda Y, Kitada M, Wakao S, et al. Unique multipotent cells in adult human mesenchymal cell populations. Proc Natl Acad Sci U S A 2010;107(19): 8639–43.

8. De Miguel MP, Fuentes-Julián S, Blázquez-Martínez A, et al. Immunosuppressive properties of mesenchymal stem cells: advances and applications. Curr Mol Med 2012;12(5):574–91.

9. Eto H, Kato H, Suga H, et al. The fate of adipocytes after non-vascularized fat grafting: evidence of early death and replacement of adipocytes. Plast Reconstr Surg 2012;129:1081–92.

10. Kato H, Mineda K, Eto H, et al. Degeneration, regeneration, and cicatrization after fat grafting: dynamic total tissue remodeling during the first three months. Plast Reconstr Surg 2014;133:303e–13e.

11. Suga H, Eto H, Shigeura T, et al. FGF-2-induced HGF secretion by adipose-derived stromal cells inhibits post-injury fibrogenesis through a JNK-dependent mechanism. Stem Cells 2009;27:238–49.

12. Doi K, Ogata F, Eto H, et al. Differential contributions of graft- and host-derived cells in tissue regeneration/remodeling after fat grafting. Plast Reconstr Surg, in press.

13. Kurita M, Matsumoto D, Shigeura T, et al. Influences of centrifugation on cells and tissues in liposuction aspirates: optimized centrifugation for lipotransfer and cell isolation. Plast Reconstr Surg 2008;121:1033–41.

14. Kim IH, Yang JD, Lee DG, et al. Evaluation of centrifugation technique and effect of epinephrine on fat cell viability in autologous fat injection. Aesthet Surg J 2009;29:35–9.

15. Zuk PA, Zhu M, Mizuno H, et al. Multilineage cells from human adipose tissue: implications for cell-based therapies. Tissue Eng 2001;7:211–28.

16. Yoshimura K, Sato K, Aoi N, et al. Cell-assisted lipotransfer (CAL) for cosmetic breast augmentation -supportive use of adipose-derived stem/stromal cells. Aesthetic Plast Surg 2008;32:48–55.

17. Yoshimura K, Sato K, Aoi N, et al. Cell-assisted lipotransfer for facial lipoatrophy: efficacy of clinical use of adipose-derived stem cells. Dermatol Surg 2008;34:1178–85.

18. Yoshimura K, Asano Y, Aoi N, et al. Progenitor-enriched adipose tissue transplantation as rescue for breast implant complications. Breast J 2010;16:169–75.

19. Sterodimas A, de Faria J, Nicaretta B, et al. Autologous fat transplantation versus adipose-derived stem cell-enriched lipografts: a study. Aesthet Surg J 2011;31:682–93.

20. Tiryaki T, Findikli N, Tiryaki D. Staged stem cell-enriched tissue (SET) injections for soft tissue augmentation in hostile recipient areas: a preliminary report. Aesthetic Plast Surg 2011;35:965–71.

21. Castro-Govea Y, De La Garza-Pineda O, Lara-Arias J, et al. Cell-assisted lipotransfer for the treatment of Parry-Romberg syndrome. Arch Plast Surg 2012;39:659–62.

22. Gentile P, Orlandi A, Scioli MG, et al. A comparative translational study: the combined use of enhanced stromal vascular fraction and platelet-rich plasma improves fat grafting maintenance in breast reconstruction. Stem Cells Transl Med 2012;1:341–51.

23. Chang Q, Li J, Dong Z, et al. Quantitative volumetric analysis of progressive hemifacial atrophy corrected using stromal vascular fraction-supplemented autologous fat grafts. Dermatol Surg 2013;39:1465–73.

24. Tanikawa DY, Aguena M, Bueno DF, et al. Fat grafts supplemented with adipose-derived stromal cells in the rehabilitation of patients with craniofacial microsomia. Plast Reconstr Surg 2013;132:141–52.

25. Gentile P, De Angelis B, Pasin M, et al. Adipose-derived stromal vascular fraction cells and platelet-rich plasma: basic and clinical evaluation for cell-based therapies in patients with scars on the face. J Craniofac Surg 2014;25:267–72.

26. Peltoniemi HH, Salmi A, Miettinen S, et al. Stem cell enrichment does not warrant a higher graft survival in lipofilling of the breast: a prospective comparative study. J Plast Reconstr Aesthet Surg 2013;66:1494–503.

27. Wang L, Luo X, Lu Y, et al. Is the resorption of grafted fat reduced in cell-assisted lipotransfer for breast augmentation? Ann Plast Surg 2014. [Epub ahead of print].

28. Kølle SF, Fischer-Nielsen A, Mathiasen AB, et al. Enrichment of autologous fat grafts with ex-vivo expanded adipose tissue-derived stem cells for graft survival: a randomised placebo-controlled trial. Lancet 2013;382:1113–20.

29. Yoshimura K, Sato K, Aoi N, et al. Ectopic fibrogenesis induced by transplantation of adipose-derived progenitor cell suspension immediately after lipoinjection. Transplantation 2008;85:1868–9.

Can We Standardize the Techniques for Fat Grafting?

Jeng-Yee Lin, MD, PhD[a], Chunmei Wang, MD, PhD[b],
Lee L.Q. Pu, MD, PhD[c],*

KEYWORDS

- Fat transplantation • Fat grafting • Lipotransfer • Coleman technique • Surgical technique

KEY POINTS

- The preferred donor sites include the low abdomen and inner thigh, especially in younger patients.
- Fat grafts should be harvested with lower negative pressure via modified liposuction technique to ensure the integrity as well as the optimal level of cellular function.
- Fat grafts should be processed with centrifugation that can reliably produce purified fat and concentrated growth factors and adipose-derived stem cells, all of which are beneficial to graft retention.
- Fat grafts should be placed following certain principles with gentle injection of a small amount per pass in multiple tissue planes and levels with multiple passes to ensure maximal contact of the graft with vascularized tissue in the recipient site.

INTRODUCTION

Fat grafting can be a good option for soft tissue augmentation because fat is abundant, readily available, inexpensive, host compatible, and can be harvested easily and repeatedly.[1] However, the overall survival rate of a fat graft is around 50% in most reported studies, which has not been considered ideal for clinical practice. The goal of improving graft retention has been, therefore, the constant driving force for scientists and clinicians to search for better techniques for fat grafting.

Refinement of fat grafting techniques has largely been investigated to maintain the fat graft's viability and to create a better environment in the recipient site for fat graft survival. In this article, the authors primarily introduce one possible preferred technique for autologous fat grafting based on the most recent scientific studies by many investigators. The authors propose it as a standardized technique because this would be a more scientifically sound approach. The authors hope the readers will be able to use the information provided here to achieve the best possible outcome of fat grafting for their patients.

CLASSIFICATIONS FOR FAT GRAFTING

The fat grafting technique can be arbitrarily classified into 5 essential components: how to select the donor sites, how to harvest the fat grafts, how to process the fat grafts, how to prepare the recipient sites, and how to inject the fat grafts. Fat grafting can also be arbitrarily divided into 3 categories based on the volume needed: Small-volume fat grafting (<100 mL) is performed primarily for facial rejuvenation or regenerative approach. Large-volume fat grafting

[a] Division of Plastic Surgery, Taipei University Hospital, Taipei, Taiwan; [b] Department of Plastic and Aesthetic Surgery, Dongguan Kanghua Hospital, Dongguan, Guangdong, China; [c] Division of Plastic Surgery, University of California Davis, 2221 Stockton Boulevard, Suite 2123, Sacramento, CA 95817, USA
* Corresponding author.
E-mail address: lee.pu@ucdmc.ucdavis.edu

Clin Plastic Surg 42 (2015) 199–208
http://dx.doi.org/10.1016/j.cps.2014.12.005
0094-1298/15/$ – see front matter © 2015 Elsevier Inc. All rights reserved.

(100–200 mL) is performed primarily for breast and body contouring. Mega-volume fat grafting (>300 mL) is performed primarily for buttock augmentation or breast augmentation or reconstruction. Each category may have its respective technique for the procedure.[2]

BASIC CONSIDERATIONS FOR FAT GRAFTING
Donor Site Selection

A variety of body areas that uniformly have abundant or excess fat are suitable as donor sites for harvest of fat grafts, such as the abdomen, flanks, buttocks, medial and lateral thighs, or knees. As a general rule, donor sites are selected that enhance the body contour and are easily accessible in the supine position, which is the position that is used for almost all facial and body augmentation procedures. Although there is no evidence of a favorable donor site for harvest of fat grafts because the viability of adipocytes within the fat grafts from different donor sites may be considered equal, a higher concentration of adipose-derived stem cells (ADSCs) is found in the lower abdomen and inner thigh in one study.[3] In addition, in a younger age group (<45 years old), fat grafts harvested from both the lower abdomen and inner thigh have higher viability based on a single assay test.[4] With what we know about the potential role of ADSCs in fat grafting,[5] the lower abdomen and inner thighs should, therefore, be chosen as the better donor sites for fat transplantation (**Fig. 1**).[3,4] These donor sites are not only easily accessible by the surgeons with patients in the supine position but also scientifically sound as long as patients have an adequate amount of adipose tissue in those areas. If patients are placed in the prone position, the posterior medial thigh, lateral thigh, and flank areas can be the primary donor sites for harvest

of more fat grafts. The palm and pinch test should be performed in the donor tissue to determine if there is adequate fat reserve and to quickly estimate the amount of fat that can be harvested.[6] A palm size is roughly measured as 200 cm^2, whereas a pinch test predicts the layer thickness of the fat graft to be harvested. For example, even in a thin patient, a 0.25-cm layer thickness of fat harvested over the surface area of a palm will yield 50 mL of fat graft (200 cm^2 × 0.25 cm = 50 mL). Therefore, we can harvest 250 mL of fat solely from the anterior surface of a woman's thigh that has 5 palm measures.

Anesthesia

Anesthesia for harvest of fat grafts can be performed under general anesthesia, epidural anesthesia, or local anesthesia with or without sedation. Intravenous sedation is routinely used in conjunction with regional or local anesthesia if requested by patients. The tumescent solution used for donor site analgesia or hemostasis should contain the lowest concentration of lidocaine possible because its high concentration may have a detrimental effect on the adipocyte function and viability.[7] In general, the authors often use 0.01% to 0.02% of lidocaine in Ringer lactate if the fat grafting procedure is performed under general anesthesia and 0.04% if the procedure is under local anesthesia with or without sedation. The tumescent solution also contains epinephrine with a concentration of 1:1,000,000. Epinephrine can precipitate vasoconstriction in the donor sites as well as the recipient sites, which may decrease blood loss, bruising, hematoma, and the possibility of intra-arterial injection of the transplanted fat, especially when injecting around periorbital areas or in the face.

Fat Graft Harvesting

The syringe aspiration, as a relatively less traumatic method for harvest of fat grafts, is supported by the more recent studies and should be considered as a standardized technique of choice for harvest of fat grafts.[8] However, this technique can be time consuming even for experienced surgeons; the large quantity of fat grafts may not be easily obtained with this technique. Several manufactures have attempted to develop an ideal device that combines the fat harvest, process, and transfer.[9] Unfortunately, only a few such devices have been studied comprehensively for their reliability; their usefulness is still debatable even among the experts in the field.[10,11]

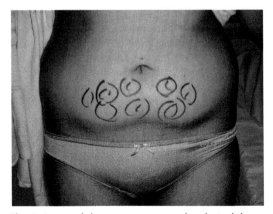

Fig. 1. Lower abdomen as a commonly selected donor site for small-volume fat grafting.

Small-volume harvesting technique

Placement of incisions can be done with a No. 11 blade in the locations where the future scar can be easily concealed. Fat grafts can be harvested through the same incision made for infiltration of the aesthetic solution. The size of the incision is about 2 to 3 mm. A tenotomy scissor is used to dilate the underlying subcutaneous tissue through the incision to allow insertion of the harvesting cannula with ease. The aesthetic solution is then infiltrated to the donor site 10 to 15 minutes before fat extraction, which makes harvesting of the fat graft easier and less traumatic. The ratio of aspirated fat to tumescent solution should be about 1:1 so that each pass of fat extraction can be more efficient.

A 10-mL Luer-Lok syringe is used and connected with a harvesting cannula. The authors prefer a 10-mL syringe to a larger one because the 10-mL syringe is less cumbersome in hand. The harvesting cannula is 15 cm long with a blunt tip and has dual openings like the shape of a bucket handle (**Fig. 2**). Gently pulling back on the plunger creates a 2-mL space vacuum of negative pressure in the syringe. With a gentle back-and-forth movement of the syringe, the fat is gradually collected inside the syringe (**Fig. 3**). If little fat with too much fluid is present within the syringe, the fluid can be easily pushed out from the bottom of the syringe in a vertical position and fat extraction can be continued. After harvest, all incision sites are closed with interrupted sutures once excess tumescent fluid or blood has been milked out.

Large- or mega-volume harvesting technique

For large-volume fat grafting, one well-conducted study has showed that fat harvested with low aspiration pressure (<250 mm Hg) has a more viable adipocyte count than that harvested with high

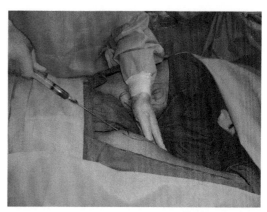

Fig. 3. Fat graft harvesting: back-and-forth movement with a 10-mL syringe, and fat grafts are easily aspirated into the syringe.

aspiration pressure (>760 mm Hg).[12] Several devices have shown their potentials for large- or mega-volume fat graft harvesting with reliability in yielding a greater number of viable adipocytes and a higher level of cellular function within fat graft compared with the standard liposuction technique. One of the examples is the LipiVage fat harvest, wash, and transfer device (Genesis Biosystems, Inc, Lewisville, TX).[9] It may have certain benefits for less-experienced surgeons to use the device for harvesting and processing fat grafts so that such fat grafts can be more consistent in terms of their viability and intact structure. Khouri and colleagues[6] advocated a low-pressure vacuum (300 mm Hg) liposuction with a specially designed device (KVAC-Syringe; Lipocosm, Key Biscayne, FL) to harvest the fat graft with constant low pressure and place it to low G force (15 g, 2 to 3 minutes) using a hand-cranked centrifugation for mega-volume graft harvest and processing. A newly designed harvesting cannula by Khouri may have many advantages because of its efficiency and less trauma to adipocytes. Such a cannula can be incorporated into a large-volume fat grafting instrument set and be used in conjunction with lower suction pressure for large-volume fat graft harvest (**Fig. 4**).

Fat Graft Processing

Several methods have been proposed to effectively remove the infiltrated solution and cell debris within the lipoaspirates and to obtain more concentrated fat grafts. However, it is actually the most controversial and disagreeable issue in fat grafting even among many experts in the field. Common methods for processing fat grafts include centrifugation, filtration, or gravity sedimentation.

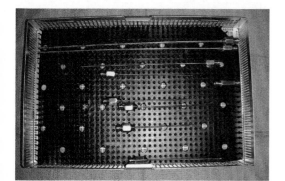

Fig. 2. The instruments used for fat injection: Different size and shape of cannulas are used as needed. The forked-tip cannula can be used to release fibrotic tissue, scar, or adhesion.

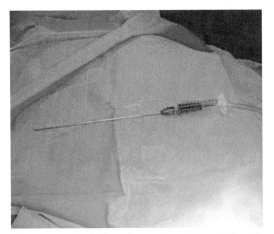

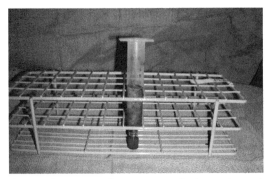

Fig. 5. The Luer-Lok aperture of the syringe is removed at completion of harvest and is ready for centrifugation.

Fig. 4. A newly designed cannula with multiple side holes for large- or mega-volume fat graft harvest.

Centrifugation, as proposed by Coleman[8], is the authors' preferred method to process fat grafts. There are several advantages of centrifugation of fat grafts. More viable adipocytes are found at the bottom of the middle layer after centrifugation even with a force of 50 g for 2 minutes based on viable cell counts, and this makes manipulation of the fat graft for use easier and with reliable viability.[13,14] Recent studies have shown that proper centrifugation can concentrate not only adipocytes and ADSCs but also several angiogenic growth factors within the processed fat grafts.[15,16] Because a higher content of stem cells or angiogenic growth factor positively correlated with fat graft survival both in experimental and clinical studies,[17] centrifugation at 3000 rpm (about 1200 g) for 3 minutes seems to offer more benefits for this effectively concentrating adipocytes and ADSCs and should be a valid method of choice for processing fat grafts, especially for small-volume fat grafting.[13]

Processing of fat with centrifugation
The Luer-Lok aperture of the 10-mL syringe locked with a plug at completion of harvest is ready for centrifugation (Fig. 5). After careful removal of the plunger, all lipoaspirate-filled 10-mL syringes are placed into a centrifuge and are then centrifuged with 3000 rpm (about 1200 g) for 3 minutes. Greater G force or longer duration of centrifugation may be harmful to adipocytes and is, therefore, not recommended.[18]

Attention should be made to avoid prolonged exposure of fat grafts to air and to avoid bacterial contamination. After being centrifuged, lipoaspirates with the syringe are divided into 3 layers: the oil content in the upper layer, fatty tissue in the middle layer, and the fluid portion at the bottom (Fig. 6). The oil can be decanted from the Luer-Lok syringe. The residual oil is wicked with a cotton strip or swab. The fluid at the bottom can be easily drained out once the plug at the Luer-Lok aperture is removed.

The concentrated fat in the syringe can then be transferred to a 1-mL syringe (the authors' preferred size of syringe for fat injection) with an adaptor (Fig. 7). A 1-mL syringe is made of acrylic material and has little resistance while fat grafts are injected. In addition, the surgeon can easily control the injected volume with such a syringe (Fig. 8). The air bubble inside the syringe should be removed; thus, quantification of the volume injected can be recorded precisely (Figs. 9 and 10).

Processing fat with the device, filtration, or gravity sedimentation
Several other fat graft processing devices (such as the Revolve system, LifeCell Corporation, Bridgewater, NJ or Puregraft, Cytori Therapeutics, Inc, San Diego, CA) that claimed to produced

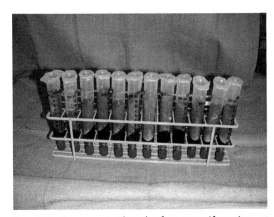

Fig. 6. Syringes are placed after centrifugation at 3000 rpm for 3 minutes. Three layers are formed: the upper layer, oil; middle layer, fat grafts; and the lower layer, liquid.

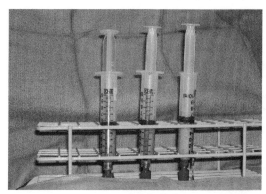

Fig. 7. After being processed, fat grafts are ready to be transferred to small syringes.

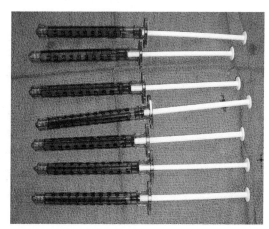

Fig. 9. A 1-mL acrylic syringe is the preferred one for small-volume fat grafting. It has little friction or resistance during the injection; therefore, the surgeon can easily control the injected volume.

equivalent or higher concentration of fat graft with reduced red blood cell (RBC) debris and free oil as compared with other alternative methods, including the Coleman technique.[10,11] These studies in fact had certain problems in experiment designs and were not tested independently. They also failed to prove its superiority in fat graft processing in terms of concentration of viability of adipocytes and in vivo graft retention rate. Several surgeons advocate the filtration technique or even just gravity sedimentation to process a large or mega volume of harvested fat grafts. However, without proper centrifugation, fat grafts processed with filtration or sedimentation may not be purely enough and contain many inflammatory materials, such as free fatty acids and fragmented RBCs. Therefore, proper centrifugation even for large- or mega-volume fat grafting can be important.

Placement of Fat Grafts

One of the most important techniques in fat grating may be how to place fat grafts. The key to a successful fat graft injection is to achieve an even distribution of fat grafts in the recipient site. By doing so, the injected fat grafts may have a maximal amount of contact with the tissue in the recipient site for better fat graft survival through plasmatic imbibition and neovascularization. Not only can grafting with a small volume in each pass get better surgical outcomes but complications, such as fibrosis, oil cyst formation, calcification or even infection with large-bolus grafting, can also be avoided. To achieve this goal, a small volume (no more than 0.1 mL) of fat grafts should be injected in each pass. Slow injection of 0.5 to 1.0 mL/s should be injected during the withdrawal phase in each pass to minimize trauma to the fat graft.[19] Fat grafts should be placed via multiple passes within multiple tissue planes and tunnels in multiple directions (**Fig. 11**).[1,20]

Injection should be as gentle as possible to avoid a possible injury to vessel or nerve. Injection with resistance would compromise the result and

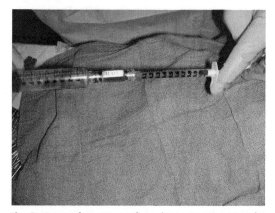

Fig. 8. Fat grafts are transferred to a 1-mL syringe for injection.

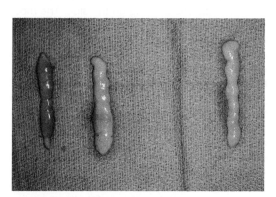

Fig. 10. An example of well-processed and concentrated fat grafts without oils and red blood cells.

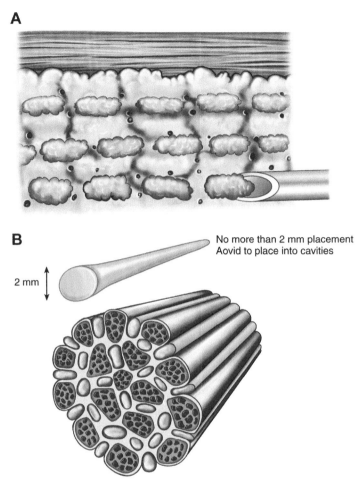

A

B

2 mm

No more than 2 mm placement
Aovid to place into cavities

Fig. 11. (*A*) A proper technique of fat injection. Placement of minuscule amounts of fat grafts with each pass as the cannula is withdrawn. Fat grafts should be placed with multiple bypasses but in multiple tissue planes and tunnels. (*B*) The placement of fat grafts within the tissue.

increase the chance of associated complications. The injecting cannulas usually range from 20 G to 12 G in diameter and vary in length and shape according to the volume and area to be grafted (see **Fig. 2**). The tip of the infiltration cannula is usually blunt and has one opening on the side. The most commonly used cannulas are 5 to 9 cm in length for facial procedures and 9 to 15 cm for body procedures. In general, a smaller cannula should be used for fat grafting to the area, such as the periorbital region, where only a smaller volume of fat grafts is injected in each pass. Small cannulas may also allow the surgeon to have more precise control over the volume when an extremely tiny amount of fat grafts is injected. The cannula includes a straight or curved one and a blunt or forked tip in order to meet different needs. The cannula with a forked tip can cut through tissues and can be used to release fibrotic tissue or scar, adhesion, or ligament attachments.

A preoperative photograph with a detail planning marked on the face of a patients is important for intraoperative comparison because the changes that need to be made with fat grafting in the operating room are usually subtle. The surgeon should make sure where the cannula tip is during the entire injection process. If there is any doubt about the tip location, tent the cannula tip toward the skin and then see blanching of the skin overlying the advanced cannula to reveal its exact location. If fat grafts are placed in a correct location, the augmented effect in the grafted area can be easily identified. If volume is not increased even though grafting is in the right place, other factors that may restrict volume enlargement should be taken into consideration, such as fibrotic adhesion, retaining ligaments, or tight skin envelope. Fibrosis or adhesion can be dissected with an 18-G needle or a forked-tip cannula. Tight skin envelope may require pre-expansion before fat grafting. For large- or mega-volume fat grafting, the principle for the placement of fat grafts should be the same as small-volume fat grafting except more volume (ie, 1 mL of fat grafts) can be injected in each pass because the recipient site is much large (see **Fig. 11**B).[6] Attention should be made to avoid a bolus injection, and the basic principles for the placement of fat grafts should be followed to ensure a better outcome and avoid fat necrosis.

Overcorrection

Whether overcorrection is necessary or not for fat grafting remains unclear. Because the viable fat grafts are only observed in the peripheral zone approximately 1.5 mm from the edge of the grafts and the percentage of graft viability depends on its thickness and geometric shape,[21] overcorrection for better graft survival in the recipient site seems to lack scientific support. In addition, significant overcorrection may increase the incidence of fat necrosis and subsequent calcification or even severe infection.[22] Therefore, significant overcorrection should be avoided until its necessity and safety can be confirmed by future studies.

Postoperative Care

Swelling in the recipient site is expected for 1 or 2 weeks, and the grafted areas can become firm or hard in the first few weeks. Patients should be informed about this normal process after fat grafting, and some reassurance to them may be necessary. However, when fat grafting is done to the face, prolonged swelling (up to 6 weeks) may be expected. During the recovery time, ice packing, tight compression with elastic bandage, or massage in the grafted area should be avoided because all of the above may compromise fat graft survival and the final outcome. However, taping over the grafted areas may relieve some discomfort from swelling and prevent patients from pressing or touching the areas (**Fig. 12**). Any direct trauma or shear force over the grafted areas may jeopardize fat graft survival and should be avoided.

Timing for Subsequent Injection

Because the overall take rate of fat grafting by even experienced surgeons ranges from 50% to 90%,[1,20,23] additional procedures are frequently necessary to achieve an optimal outcome. However, there is no scientific study that has addressed the timing of subsequent fat grafting. So far, only expert opinion has been mentioned in the literature regarding this specific issue. It has been suggested that the timing of additional fat grafting sessions should be deferred until 6 months postoperatively to diminish the "inflammatory response" in the grafted area.[24]

It is often difficult to assess the surgical outcome during the first few weeks after fat grafting. In general, the extent of swelling and the waiting period that it needs to resolve is also volume dependent. The authors have observed the transplanted fat gradually loses its volume with time and usually becomes stabilized at 3 months postoperatively if surgical recovery is uneventful. Therefore, the timing of a subsequent fat grafting procedure should be deferred to at least 3 months after previous transplantation.

NEW CONCEPTS OR METHODS FOR FAT GRAFTING

Several novel concepts and technologies have been introduced to improve graft survival and retention after fat grafting. Each new treatment has its rationale based on improvement of one or

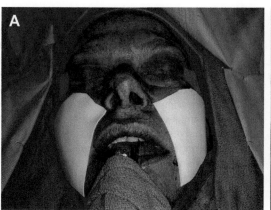
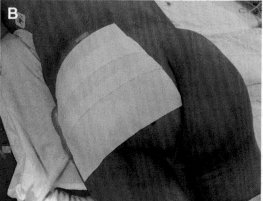

Fig. 12. Taping the injected area for immediate postoperative care after fat grafting. (*A*) After small-volume facial fat grafting; (*B*) After large-volume fat grafting for buttock augmentation.

Table 1
Potential novel treatments for improvement of fat graft retention

	Mechanism	Clinical Relevance
ADSCs	Regenerate adipocytes in the fat graft and promote neovascularization into the fat graft	The safety and efficacy not yet determined
SVF	Potentially regenerates adipocytes in the graft and promotes neovascularization in the fat graft	Clinically feasible; the efficacy not yet determined
EVE	Increase tissue thickness, promotes angiogenesis, and activates resident progenitor cells in the recipient sites	Clinically feasible; effectiveness probably device and patient-compliance dependent

Abbreviations: EVE, external volume expansion; SVF, stromal vascular fraction.

more of the following processes: fat harvest, processing, injection, or preparation of the recipient site (**Table 1**).

Use of Adipose-Derived Stem Cells

Higher ADSCs content correlates positively with improved fat graft retention in both experimental and clinical studies. Improvement of fat graft retention is probably through regeneration of the adipocytes within the fat graft construct by ADSCs, which obtain self-renewal capacity.[17] The safety issue and efficacy regarding the use of ADSCs in fat grafting are not yet determined and, therefore, need more investigations before it can be put into clinical practice. Instead, cell-assisted lipotransfer as proposed by Yoshimura and colleagues[25] using stromal vascular fraction (SVF), which contain a heterogeneous group of cells including ADSCs, blood-derived cells (CD45+), endothelial (progenitor) cells, and pericytes, is imminent and practically available.[25] It is hypothesized that augmentation of the fat graft with SVF can improved fat graft retention by increasing angiogenesis and regeneration of adipocytes in the graft. However, more randomized clinical trials should be conducted to prove its benefits in fat graft survival.

Preparation of Recipient Sites with External Volume Expansion

Preparation of the recipient site as a better environment for the fat graft to survive is another important factor of increasing graft retention after fat grafting. One innovative way of achieving this goal first proposed by Khouri and colleagues[26] is pre-expansion of the recipient site using an external device to apply a continued negative pressure on the recipient site skin, no different from the vacuum therapy used in promotion of wound healing. Because high graft retention is most critical and difficult to achieve in mega-volume fat grafting, such as in cases of breast augmentation or reconstruction, a specially designed external pre-expansion device for the breast was first used in fat grafting to the breast. This pre-expansion device or external volume expansion (EVE) for the breast was proved successful in increasing long-term fat retention in the breast based on scientific studies. Khouri and colleagues[26] hypothesized that EVE may potentially increase the thickness of tissue and improve angiogenesis in the recipient site. It was also reported that EVE induces adipose tissue enlargement by activating resident progenitor cells combined with controlled release of basic fibroblast growth factor as well as with vascular remodeling.[27,28] Lancerotto and colleagues[29] found that EVE induces mechanical stimulation, edema, ischemia, and inflammation in the recipient site, thus, maintaining an environment conducive to cell proliferation and angiogenesis over distinct time periods. Disadvantages of the use of EVE include patient commitment and compliance to its continued and uninterrupted use, skin rashes, dermatitis, and postinflammatory hyperpigmentation.

SUMMARY

Much of the current scientific studies support the authors' preferred fat grafting technique described in this article for small-volume fat grafting, and that can be standardized.[30] However, the techniques for large- or mega-volume fat grafting have not been standardized yet. Besides the proper selection of donor sites (ie, the lower abdomen or inner thigh for small-volume fat grafting), fat grafts should be harvested with a less traumatic method, such as syringe aspiration or lower suction pressure, and then processed with proper centrifugation. Fat grafts should be placed in a small amount (no more than 0.1 mL or equivalent amount for large volume) for each pass but with multiple passes in multiple tunnels, multiple tissue levels, and multiple directions. Anesthetic (or

Table 2
Summary of basic considerations and techniques for fat grafting

Preferred donor sites	Lower abdomen or inner thigh
Anesthesia	Low concentration of lidocaine for infiltration
Fat graft harvesting	A less traumatic syringe technique or lower pressure suction technique
Fat graft processing	Centrifugation with a proper setting (ie, 3000 rpm or 1200 g for 3 min)
Recipient site preparation (for large or mega volume)	Use of EVE device to improve vascularity and adipogenesis
Placement of fat grafts	Placed in a small amount (0.1 mL or equivalent amount) for each pass in the withdraw phase but with multiple passes in multiple tissue planes, multiple levels, and multiple directions
Overcorrection	Not recommended
Postoperative care	Proper mobilization of the grafted area Swelling always expected Additional injection may be necessary
Timing for subsequent injection	3–6 mo after previous injection

tumescent) solution with a low lidocaine concentration should be chosen for infiltration of the donor site. Significant overcorrection should be avoided to minimize complications, such as fat necrosis. The timing for subsequent injection may be about 3 to 6 months after previous injection (**Table 2**). It is also critical to inform patients that a subsequent procedure may be necessary after the first fat grafting if the expected results have not been achieved.

REFERENCES

1. Coleman SR. Structural fat grafting: more than a permanent filler. Plast Reconstr Surg 2006;118: 108S–20S.
2. Del Vecchio D, Rohrich RJ. A classification of clinical fat grafting: different problems, different solutions. Plast Reconstr Surg 2012;130:511–22.
3. Padoin AV, Braga-Silva J, Martins P, et al. Sources of processed lipoaspirate cells: influence of donor site on cell concentration. Plast Reconstr Surg 2008;122: 614–8.
4. Geissler PJ, Davis K, Roostaeian J, et al. Improving fat transfer viability: the role of aging, body mass index, and harvest site. Plast Reconstr Surg 2014;134: 227–32.
5. Yoshimura K, Suga H, Eto H. Adipose-derived stem/progenitor cells: roles in adipose tissue remodeling and potential use for soft tissue augmentation. Regen Med 2009;4:265–73.
6. Khouri RK, Rigotti G, Cardoso E, et al. Megavolume autologous fat transfer: part II. Practice and techniques. Plast Reconstr Surg 2014;133:1369–77.
7. Keck M, Zeyda M, Gollinger K, et al. Local anesthetics have a major impact on viability of preadipocytes and their differentiation into adipocytes. Plast Reconstr Surg 2010;123:1500–5.
8. Pu LL, Coleman SR, Cui X, et al. Autologous fat grafts harvested and refined by the Coleman technique: a comparative study. Plast Reconstr Surg 2008;122:932–7.
9. Ferguson RE, Cui X, Fink BF, et al. The viability of autologous fat grafts harvested with the LipiVage system: a comparative study. Ann Plast Surg 2008;60:594–7.
10. Ansorge H, Garza JR, McCormack MC, et al. Autologous fat processing via Revolve system: quality and quantity of fat retention evaluated in an animal model. Aesthet Surg J 2014;34:438–47.
11. Zhu M, Cohen SR, Hicok KC, et al. Comparison of three different fat graft preparation methods: gravity separation, centrifugation, and simultaneous washing with filtration in a closed system. Plast Reconstr Surg 2013;131:873–80.
12. Cheriyan T, Kao HK, Qiao X, et al. Low harvest pressure enhances autologous fat graft viability. Plast Reconstr Surg 2014;133:1365–8.
13. Boscher MT, BeCkert BW, Puckett CL, et al. Analysis of lipocyte viability after liposuction. Plast Reconstr Surg 2002;109:761–5.
14. Pu LL, Cui X, Fink BF, et al. The viability of fatty tissues within adipose aspirates after conventional liposuction: a comprehensive study. Ann Plast Surg 2005;54:288–92.
15. Kurita M, Matsumoto D, Shigeura T, et al. Influences of centrifugation on cells and tissues in liposuction aspirates: optimized centrifugation for lipotransfer and cell isolation. Plast Reconstr Surg 2008;121:1033–41.
16. Pallua N, Pulsfort AK, Suschek C, et al. Content of the growth factors bFGF, IGF-1, VEGF, and PDGF-BB in freshly harvested lipoaspirate after centrifugation and incubation. Plast Reconstr Surg 2009;123:826–33.

17. Philips BJ, Grahovac TL, Valentin JE, et al. Prevalence of endogenous CD34+ adipose stem cells predicts human fat graft retention in a xenograft model. Plast Reconstr Surg 2013;132:845–58.

18. Kim IH, Yang JD, Lee DG, et al. Evaluation of centrifugation technique and effect of epinephrine on fat cell viability in autologous fat injection. Aesthet Surg J 2009;29:35–9.

19. Lee JH, Kirkham JC, McCormack MC, et al. The effect of pressure and shear on autologous fat grafting. Plast Reconstr Surg 2013;131:1125–36.

20. Xie Y, Zheng DN, Li QF, et al. An integrated fat grafting technique for cosmetic facial contouring. J Plast Reconstr Aesthet Surg 2010;63:270–6.

21. Carpaneda CA, Ribeiro MT. Percentage of graft viability versus injected volume in adipose autotransplants. Aesthet Plast Surg 1994;18:17–9.

22. Sherman JE, Fanzio PM, White H, et al. Blindness and necrotizing fasciitis after liposuction and fat transfer. Plast Reconstr Surg 2010;126:1358–63.

23. Gutowski CA. Current applications and safety of autologous fat grafts: a report of the ASPS fat graft task force. Plast Reconstr Surg 2009;124:272–80.

24. Kanchwala SK, Glatt BS, Conant EF, et al. Autologous fat grafting to the reconstructed breast: the management of acquired contour deformities. Plast Reconstr Surg 2009;124:409–18.

25. Yoshimura K, Katsujiro S, Noriyuki A, et al. Cell-assisted lipotransfer for cosmetic breast augmentation: supportive use of adipose-derived stem/stromal cells. Aesthet Plast Surg 2008;32:48–55.

26. Khouri RK, Eisenmann KM, Cardoso E, et al. Brava and autologous fat transfer is a safe and effective breast augmentation alternative: results of a 6-year, 81 patient, prospective multicenter study. Plast Reconstr Surg 2012;129:1173–87.

27. Kato H, Suga H, Eto H, et al. Reversible adipose tissue enlargement induced by external tissue suspension: possible contribution of basic fibroblast growth factor in the preservation of enlarged tissue. Tissue Eng Part A 2010;16:2029–40.

28. Heit YI, Lancerotto L, Mesteri I, et al. External volume expansion increases subcutaneous thickness, cell proliferation, and vascular remodeling in a murine model. Plast Reconstr Surg 2012;130:541–7.

29. Lancerotto L, Chin MS, Freniere B, et al. Mechanism of action of external volume expansion devices. Plast Reconstr Surg 2013;132:569–78.

30. Pu LL. Towards more rationalized approach to autologous fat grafting. J Plast Reconstr Aesthet Surg 2012;65:413–9.

Update on Cryopreservation of Adipose Tissue and Adipose-derived Stem Cells

Zhiquan Shu, PhD[a], Dayong Gao, PhD[a],
Lee L.Q. Pu, MD, PhD[b],*

KEYWORDS

- Cryopreservation • Adipose cells • Adipose tissue • Adipose-derived stem cells (ADSCs)

KEY POINTS

- Controlled slow freezing (1–2°C/min) and fast thawing together with a combination of cryoprotective agents (CPAs) shows optimal results.
- Adipose-derived stem cells (ADSCs), either isolated from fresh adipose tissues before ADSC cryopreservation or isolated from cryopreserved adipose tissue, can retain their proliferation and differentiation capabilities after cryopreservation. This property ensures the probability of ADSCs serving as an important source for cell-based therapy and tissue engineering.
- Future work for cryopreservation of adipose tissue includes development of novel cryoprotection media (DMSO free, serum free, and even xeno free), fundamental cryobiological studies of adipose tissue and ADSCs, optimization and standardization of fat cryopreservation protocols toward good manufacturing practice products.

INTRODUCTION

One main obstacle to achieve long-term favorable results of soft tissue filling with autologous fat transplantation is the high absorption rate of the injected fat in the grafted site, reaching up to 70% of its volume.[1] Some dead materials and insufficient revascularization in the grafts are probably responsible for this problem over time.[2] This high absorption rate necessitates overcorrection and reinjection procedures in the desired area, which are associated with repeated suction-assisted lipectomy operations to obtain the fat, as well as higher cost, unfavorable appearance, increasing patient morbidity, and discomfort. In order to solve this problem, long-term cryopreservation of the

obtained fat is indispensable for both surgeons and patients. Adipose cells and tissues obtained from only a single harvest can be stored and used for the multiple grafting sessions in the future, therefore significantly reducing the patient discomfort, morbidity, cost, and time. Some researchers have also reported that transplantation of frozen fat caused less swelling and discoloration than fresh fat in the operation area.[3,4]

Another fact that necessitates cryopreservation of adipose tissues is that adipose tissue is an ideal source of many cell types, including adipocytes, preadipocytes, vascular endothelial cells, vascular smooth muscle cells, and adipose tissue–derived stem cells. These stem cells can be differentiated with specific growth factors into multiple lineages,

Disclosure: The authors declare no competing financial interests.
[a] Department of Mechanical Engineering, University of Washington, Seattle, WA 98195, USA; [b] Division of Plastic Surgery, University of California Davis, 2221 Stockton Boulevard, Suite 2123, Sacramento, CA 95817, USA
* Corresponding author.
E-mail address: lee.pu@ucdmc.ucdavis.edu

Clin Plastic Surg 42 (2015) 209–218
http://dx.doi.org/10.1016/j.cps.2014.12.001

such as fat, bone, cartilage, skeletal, muscle, endothelium, hematopoietic cells, hepatocytes, and neuronal cells. Hence, they have immeasurable applications in regenerative medicine and tissue engineering. When a cellular therapy is needed, previously cryopreserved adipose tissues can be processed in vitro to obtain such cell types for patients. Cryopreservation of adipose tissues can provide an abundant source for the ready availability of such cell types. It also serves several other purposes, including sample shipment, quality assay, donor-recipient matching, disease screening, and pooling of samples obtained from multiple procedures to get a large enough dose for clinical treatment.

Despite its advantages and significance, cryopreservation can also be a notable variable in fat processing, which may lead to viability and functionality loss of cells and tissues after freezing and thawing. There has been a lot of work conducted in the last decade to investigate and optimize the cryopreservation protocols for fat cells, tissues, and adipose tissue–derived stem cells (ADSCs).[2,4–32] Inconsistent or even opposite results can be found in the literature. Therefore, cryopreservation of adipose cells and tissues is updated in this article, starting with some fundamentals of cryobiology and cryopreservation. Then, progress in cryopreservation of adipose tissues and ADSCs is reviewed, followed by discussion of future work.

FUNDAMENTAL CRYOBIOLOGY AND CRYOPRESERVATION PROCESSES
Freezing of Cells

Optimization of isolated cell cryopreservation requires a quantitative understanding of the biophysical response of cells during the freezing process. As cells are cooled to a subzero temperature, such as about $-5°C$, both the cells and surrounding medium usually remain unfrozen despite the temperature having fallen below the freezing point of water (a supercooled state). Between $-5°C$ and about $-15°C$, ice forms in the external medium but the cell contents remain unfrozen and supercooled, presumably because the plasma membrane blocks the growth of ice crystals into the cytoplasm. The supercooled water in the cells has, by definition, a higher chemical potential than that of water in the partially frozen extracellular solution, and thus water flows out of the cell and freezes externally.

The subsequent physical events in the cell depend on the cooling rate. These cell responses to freezing were first expressed quantitatively by Mazur[33] and directly linked with cell cryoinjury by

Mazur's 2-factor hypothesis: (1) at slow cooling rates, cryoinjury occurs because of a solution effect (ie, the intracellular solute/electrolyte concentration increases as water leaves the cell, to a point at which severe cell dehydration occurs); and (2) at high cooling rates, water is not lost fast enough and cryoinjury occurs because of intracellular ice formation (IIF), which ruptures the cell membrane. The optimal cooling rate for cell survival should be slow enough to reduce IIF but fast enough to minimize the solution effects. The freezing behavior of the cells can be modified by the addition of cryoprotective agents (CPAs), which affect the rates of water transport, ice nucleation, and ice crystal growth.

More detailed information about cryobiology can be found in a review published in 1970 by Mazur[34] in *Science*. Important milestones in cryobiology since then have been the development of cryomicroscopy, allowing the observation of cell behavior during freezing and thawing[35]; devices to model and measure cell membrane permeabilities[36,37]; and mathematical modeling to describe the probability of IIF as a function of cooling rate, temperature, and cell type.[38] Karlsson and colleagues[39] incorporated into these models the effect of CPA addition on IIF formation and successfully predicted IIF formation as a function of cooling rate, temperature and CPA concentration, leading to optimal cooling protocols preventing IIF.

Thawing of Cells

Cells that have survived cooling to low temperatures still face the challenges of thawing, which can exert effects on survival comparable with those of cooling.[34] The effects depend on whether the prior rate of cooling has induced intracellular freezing or cell dehydration. In the former case, rapid thawing can rescue many cells, possibly because it can prevent the harmful growth of small intracellular ice crystals into larger crystals by recrystallization.

Addition and Removal of Cryoprotective Agents

Cells require equilibration with molar concentrations of CPAs to survive freezing. However, these CPAs have dramatic osmotic effects on cells. Cells exposed to molar concentrations of permeating CPAs undergo extensive initial dehydration followed by rehydration and potential gross swelling when the CPAs are removed. Unless precautions are taken, this shrinkage and/or swelling can be extensively enough to cause cell damage and death. Knowledge of cell membrane permeability to water and CPAs allows the prediction of the minimal and maximal cell volume excursions during addition and removal of CPAs, providing a quantitative optimization approach (eg, stepwise increase or decrease of CPA concentration in cells or tissues) to avoid osmotic damage.[40]

Fig. 1 shows the general process, cellular injury mechanisms, and optimization work for cell cryopreservation.

Cryopreservation of Whole Tissue

It is important to emphasize that successful cryopreservation of tissues is not a simple matter of extrapolating the well-established principles of cell cryopreservation to more complex tissues. Multicellular tissues are more complex than single cells, both structurally and functionally, and this is reflected in their requirements for cryopreservation. Successful cryopreservation of individual cells in the tissues is necessary, but not sufficient, for the successful cryopreservation of tissues. More than cell survival, complete structural integrity and function retention are vital for tissue cryopreservation.

Cryopreservation of complex tissues adds a set of additional problems to the known mechanisms of cryoinjury that apply to single cells in suspensions[41]:

1. Extracellular ice formation presents a major hazard for cryopreservation of multicellular tissues. The amount and location of extracellular ice affects the postthaw function of tissues. As a result, ice formation needs to be limited, restricted to harmless sites, or even totally prevented (which leads to the significance of vitrification).
2. Vascular damage or rupture is caused by ice formation/expansion in capillaries and blood vessels. The rupture of capillaries by accumulating ice explains the deleterious effect of extracellular ice in severely damaged tissues. To minimize this cryodestructive effect, a better understanding of the fundamental mechanisms of ice formation and cell dehydration in tissues is required. Although these biophysical events have been extensively studied in single cells using cryomicroscopy, similar experimental data in whole tissues are still lacking.

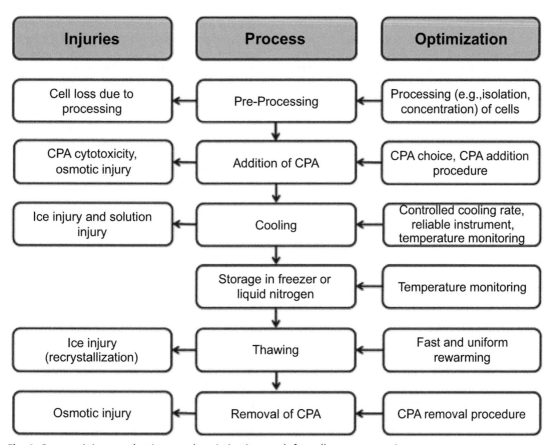

Fig. 1. Process, injury mechanisms, and optimization work for cell cryopreservation.

3. Thermal stress during the warming process causes frozen tissues to crack or fracture. Thermal stress is one type of mechanical stress caused by nonuniform heating in a frozen body, which can be reduced by uniform heating. However, because biological tissues have low thermal conductivities, high specific heats, and large volumes, conventional heating methods (eg, heating in a stirred water bath) cause large temperature gradients within the tissue, leading to high thermal stress and tissue fracture, especially for tissue with large volumes.

CRYOPRESERVATION OF ADIPOSE TISSUE

Prior studies on the viability of cryopreserved fat tissues have shown a wide range of results, which were even contradictory and continuously in debate. For example, it was reported that no or very few harmful effects were generated on the fat samples cryopreserved at −20°C without controlling of the cooling process and even without CPA, and live adipocytes were found after preservation at this temperature.[5,6] However, this opinion was questioned by many researchers. The adipocytes were destroyed after short-term freezing at −20°C and the transplantation of adipose tissues cryopreserved at −20°C provided an injection of mostly dead cells,[2] which had no advantage compared with inert fillers and should be avoided.[8] This may be one reason for the higher rate of volume adsorption after surgery when cryopreserved fat is transplanted.[12,30] For another example, the procedures for fat cryopreservation were not well documented, or varied significantly in the literature. In most reports, scientific details of the cooling and thawing processes (eg, cooling/thawing rates, temperature, and processing time) were not provided. Some researchers provided different protocols from those that were used in their studies. Butterwick and colleagues[4] found that fast freezing to −40°C and slow thawing over a couple of hours at room temperature for fat resulted in comparable effects with fresh fat transplantation for hand surgery. After a series of comparison experiments, Pu and Cui and colleagues[7,9,11–14,18,21–23] concluded that controlled slow cooling (1–2°C/min from 22°C to −30°C) followed by transferring into liquid nitrogen, and fast thawing by stirring in a 37°C water bath until thoroughly thawed, led to the best results.

These results seem contradicting and confusing. However, they may be explained by a few uncertainties in the research reports. First, the viability and functionality of adipose cells and tissues after cryopreservation and transplantation can be affected by many variables, such as the methods of fat harvest, processing, storage, and injection;

recipient and donor sites; pretreatment of fat tissues with cell culture medium or growth factors before transplantation; correction volumes; grafting intervals; and the instrument used.[3,8,23,24] For cryopreservation, variables include CPA type and concentration, addition and removal of CPA (operation procedure, temperature, and duration), cooling and thawing protocols (temperatures, cooling, and thawing rates), storage temperature, and duration. Any change in these variables can contribute to the difference in results and make it difficult to compare studies. However, most reports failed to provide scientific details of these parameters. For example, cooling rate is the vital factor in cryopreservation and can lead to life or death for the cells and tissues. The cooling rate of biosamples depends on the cooling device, protocol, sample container, and sample volume. The best way to investigate the freezing process is to directly measure the temperature change profile in dummy samples during the whole process with temperature meters, which is also necessary for better quality control toward good manufacturing practice (GMP) products. However, this information was omitted in most studies.

The second uncertainty in the different studies is the methods used for the cell/tissue viability and functionality assessments. So far, several methods have been applied in the literature to assess adipose cells and tissues, which can be classified by cell membrane integrity assays; cell functional assays and tissue assessments, including extracellular glycerol-3-phosphate dehydrogenase assessment; trypan blue and flavin adenine dinucleotide/ethidium bromide for cell membrane integrity; 3-(4,5-dimethylthiazol-2-yl)-2,5-diphenyltetrazolium bromide (MTT) and 2,3-bis-(2-Methoxy-4-nitro-5-sulfophenyl)-2H-tetrazolium (XTT) for mitochondrial activity, using cell surface markers to identify survived transplanted cells; histology; and weight and volume study for tissue evaluation.[2,3,5,6,9,13,23,24,27] Different methods and different personnel may generate different results and conclusions. Some staining techniques like Trypan blue are recognized as inaccurate because mature adipocytes contain scant cytoplasm. Dead cells without nuclei or mitochondrial activity may be interpreted as live cells when the shapes of the cells appear normal under the microscope.[3,8,24,29] All these factors also make it difficult to compare different studies.

Another significant variable in the literature for adipose cryopreservation is the CPA used. Besides the most widely used CPA, DMSO, many other kinds of CPAs were investigated for adipose cryopreservation in the last decade, including permeable and nonpermeable ones, such as glycerol, trehalose, sucrose, hydroxyethyl starch (HES), polyvinyl pyridine (PVP), and dextran.[2,7,9,13,22,27,42] In spite of few reports claiming no or even negative effects of CPAs,[6] most studies agreed that CPAs were needed for optimal cryopreservation of fat. Permeable and nonpermeable CPAs play their roles in cryoprotection with different mechanisms. A permeable CPA, like DMSO, is thought to protect cells against freezing injury by reducing ice formation inside and outside the cells. It can also penetrate into cells, fill the intracellular space, and prevent severe cell shrinkage during cell dehydration (water transport across cell membrane). Nonpermeable CPAs, like trehalose and HES, may provide protection in several ways. They dehydrate cells, thus reducing the amount of intracellular water before freezing. They also enhance the vitrification tendency of the solution, and stabilize cell membranes and proteins during freezing and drying.[7,41,43] It was found that trehalose alone or together with DMSO at reduced concentration provided comparable cryoprotection in adipose cryopreservation.[7,9,12,13,18,21–23] Besides the mechanisms mentioned earlier, the special cryoprotection function of trehalose may be related to its unique properties. As a type of disaccharide, trehalose has a large hydration radius (about 2.5 times that of other common sugars) and distinctly higher glass transition temperature than other sugars, and so can function better to keep the cell membrane intact after dehydration, facilitate the ion transport through the membrane, decrease the melting point of the membrane lipids, maximize the stability of proteins, and prevent injury to membranes caused by membrane phase transition.[44] Therefore, more extensive studies are needed on the cryoprotection function of trehalose for adipose cells and tissues.

DMSO can protect cells from cryoinjury; however, it is also cytotoxic, especially at high temperatures (such as room temperature or human body temperature). Infusion of frozen-thawed cellular products together with DMSO has been associated with several types of adverse reaction, ranging from mild events like nausea/vomiting, hypotension or hypertension, abdominal cramps, diarrhea, and flushing and chills to more severe life-threatening events like cardiac arrhythmia, encephalopathy, acute renal failure, and respiratory depression.[45] Hence, it is preferable for DMSO to be removed before the infusion. Removal of DMSO can cause cell loss caused by osmotic injury and clumping; in addition, it is time consuming, needs special equipment and expertise, and may introduce contamination during processing. Thus, cryopreservation media with reduced DMSO concentration, or even a DMSO-free alternative CPA, are desirable. Pu and colleagues[7,9,12,21,23] found that, by using optimized freezing and thawing protocols, trehalose plus DMSO at reduced concentration, or even trehalose alone, could provide comparable results for adipose tissue cryopreservation (**Fig. 2**). Further progress will increase the clinical applications of fat transplantation.

Table 1 shows the recommended method for cryopreservation of adipose tissue.

CRYOPRESERVATION OF ADIPOSE-DERIVED STEM CELLS

Adipose tissue has been found to be an important source of human adult stem cells for possible

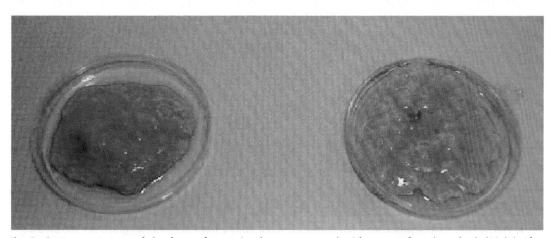

Fig. 2. Gross appearance of the fat grafts previously cryopreserved with our preferred method. (*Right*) After thawing, the fats have a near-normal appearance, much like that of freshly aspirated/refined fat grafts (*left*), and may readily be used for future fat grafting in patients if indicated. (*From* Pu LL. Cryopreservation of adipose tissue for fat grafting: problems and solutions. In: Coleman SR, Mazzola RF, editors. Fat injection: from filling to regeneration. St Louis (MO): Quality Medical Publishing; 2009. p. 84; with permission.)

Table 1
Recommended protocol for cryopreservation of adipose tissue

Procedures	Recommended Protocol	Comments
CPA selection	• Combination of permeable and non-permeable CPAs; eg, 0.5 M DMSO + 0.2 M trehalose	• Lower DMSO concentration leads to lower cytotoxicity • DMSO-free cryomedia are needed
CPA addition	• Add CPA stock solution (precooled at 4°C, 2× concentration) to adipose tissue stepwise at 4°C or room temperature (with final volume ratio 1:1) • Equilibration for no more than 30 min	• Slow addition can reduce cell volume excursion and osmotic injury • Lower temperature may reduce CPA cytotoxicity, but reduce the CPA diffusion in tissue as well
Cooling	• Controlled slow cooling to a temperature (eg, −35°C) at 1–2°C/min • Equilibration for about 10 min • Put into −80°C freezer or liquid nitrogen	• Slow cooling is needed to reduce ice injury to cells • Temperature recording in whole process is recommended
Storage	• Storage in −80°C freezer or liquid nitrogen	• −80°C for storage for months • Liquid nitrogen for storage for years • Temperature monitoring in whole process is recommended
Thawing	• Fast thawing by stirring in 37°C water bath until thoroughly thawed	• Fast thawing is beneficial to reduce recrystallization and ice injury
CPA removal	• Add isotonic medium slowly to fat tissue followed by equilibration and washing • Repeated dilution/washing may be needed	• Slow removal can reduce cell volume excursion and osmotic injury

cell-directed therapy or tissue engineering because of its advantages, such as being an abundant source, similarities with bone marrow in terms of embryonic origin, and easy availability through liposuction.[18,21] There are 2 strategies for cell-based tissue engineering and transplantation with adipose-derived stem cells (ADSCs): (1) processing the adipose tissue to obtain the stem cells and preserving the stem cells; and (2) preserving the adipose tissues until stem cell processing (**Fig. 3**).[21]

These different strategies lead to different methods of cryopreservation: cell freezing or tissue freezing, which have common but distinct scientific problems, as mentioned earlier. Both strategies have been reported in the literature and have achieved success. Wang and colleagues[29] and Choudhery and colleagues[31] found that the capabilities of ADSC proliferation and differentiation were well maintained after isolation from cryopreserved adipose tissues. Cryopreserved fat tissues can

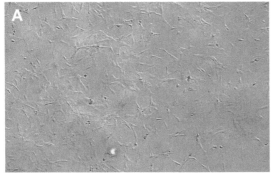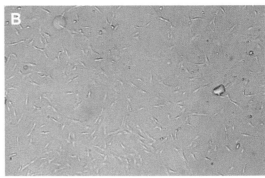

Fig. 3. Flat, spindle-shaped processed ADSCs after a 2-week culture from the fresh fat grafts are shown (*A*) and from the previously cryopreserved fat grafts (*B*). Phase-contrast microscopy was used with an original magnification of 100×. Both ADSCs appear to have normal morphology and may be used for cell-based therapy in the future. (*From* Pu LL. Cryopreservation of adipose tissue for fat grafting: problems and solutions. In: Coleman SR, Mazzola RF, editors. Fat injection: from filling to regeneration. St Louis (MO): Quality Medical Publishing; 2009. p. 75; with permission.)

serve as an alternative source of ADSCs to fresh tissues.[31] In contrast, isolated ADSCs from fresh fat tissues, including human, mouse, and equine, were also successfully cryopreserved with retained potency of proliferation and differentiation into adipocytes, osteoblasts, and chondrocytes.[15–17,19,20,25,26,28,32,46] **Table 2** shows the current optimal method for cryopreservation of ADSC, which is similar to the cryopreservation of adipose tissue shown in **Table 1**.

Adipose transfer for soft tissue augmentation may eventually be replaced by ADSC transfer because of the smaller sample volume for storage and easier cryopreservation techniques for cells compared with tissues. ADSCs are easy to grow and expand extensively in culture. ADSC transfer would be an ideal option for very thin patients with inadequate fat stores.[8] It was also reported that mesenchymal stem cells derived from adipose tissues were more robust than those from bone marrow and dental pulp.[47] The success of ADSC cryopreservation ensures the availability of autologous banked ADSCs for clinical applications in the future.[16]

FUTURE PERSPECTIVES

From the viewpoint of cryobiology and cryopreservation, some important work is needed to increase the applications of fat transplantation in the future, which includes:

1. Development of novel, DMSO-free, serum-free, or even xeno-free cryoprotection media for the cryopreservation of adipose cells and tissues. This effort will address all the problems posed by the presence of DMSO, which introduces a potentially dangerous animal serum and xeno-component to the recipient after fat transplantation. Thirumala and colleagues[25] showed the feasibility of serum-free media with reduced DMSO concentration for ADSC cryopreservation. Schulz and colleagues[48,49] showed some important progress toward a xeno-free, chemically defined cryopreservation medium for peripheral blood mononuclear cells, which can also be helpful for the optimization of adipose cryopreservation.

2. Fundamental cryobiological studies of adipose cells and tissues for the optimization of cryopreservation protocols. The optimal cryopreservation protocol is cell/tissue type dependent, which is determined by the cell/tissue cryobiological characteristics, such as cell membrane permeability to water and CPA, osmotically inactive cell volume, cell volume osmotic tolerance limits, and heat and mass

Table 2
Recommended protocol for cryopreservation of ADSCs

Procedures	Recommended Protocol	Comments
CPA selection	• Combination of permeable and non-permeable CPAs (such as DMSO, HES, PVP) in serum-free medium	• DMSO-free, serum-free, or xeno-free chemically defined cryomedia are needed
CPA addition	• Add CPA stock solution (precooled at 4°C, 2× concentration) to ADSC suspension stepwise at 4°C (with final volume ratio 1:1) • Equilibration for no more than 15 min	• Slow addition can reduce cell volume excursion and osmotic injury • Lower temperature can reduce CPA cytotoxicity
Cooling	• Controlled slow cooling to a low temperature (eg, −35°C) at 1°C/min • Put into −80°C freezer or liquid nitrogen	• Slow cooling to reduce ice injury to cells • Temperature recording in whole process is recommended
Storage	• Storage in −80°C freezer or liquid nitrogen	• −80°C for storage for months • Liquid nitrogen for storage for years • Temperature monitoring in whole process is recommended
Thawing	• Fast thawing by stirring in 37°C water bath until thoroughly thawed	• Fast thawing to reduce recrystallization and ice injury
CPA removal	• Add isotonic medium slowly to ADSC followed by centrifugation and removal • Repeated dilution/washing may be needed	• Slow removal can reduce cell volume excursion and osmotic injury

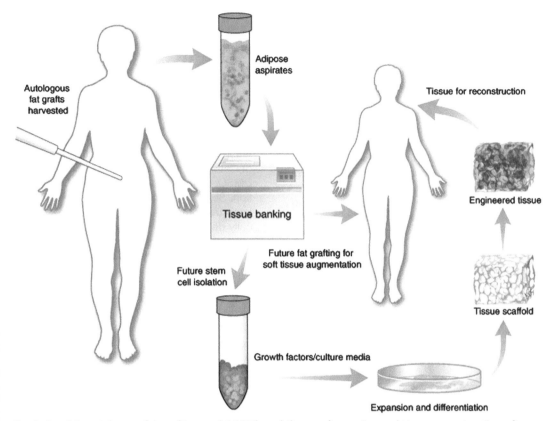

Fig. 4. Possible autologous fat grafting and ADSC-based therapy for engineered tissue reconstruction after successful cryopreservation of the patient's own adipose tissue collected from liposuction. (*From* Pu LL. Cryopreservation of adipose tissue for fat grafting: problems and solutions. In: Coleman SR, Mazzola RF, editors. Fat injection: from filling to regeneration. St Louis (MO): Quality Medical Publishing; 2009. p. 85; with permission.)

transfer properties in tissues. So far, most of the research in adipose cryopreservation has been based on empirical or semiempirical experimental design involving trial and error. Obtaining such cryobiological properties by collaboration between surgeons and cryobiologists would result in more thorough and scientific study of adipose cryopreservation.

3. Optimization and standardization of cryopreservation protocols for adipose cells and tissues. Optimization of adipose cryopreservation is still needed, including CPA selection, CPA addition and removal, cooling and thawing, and storage. Development of simple, reliable, and cost-effective devices that can be used at field sites are also greatly needed. All the processing steps should be standardized, including quality control applied through all the procedures (eg, temperature recording of samples). Other issues, including detailed labeling of specimens, informed consent, and protection of patient privacy, should also be emphasized.

SUMMARY

Despite significantly varied procedures and results in the literature for adipose cryopreservation, controlled slow freezing and fast thawing together with a combination of CPAs (including permeable and nonpermeable CPAs) showed optimal results. ADSCs, either isolated from fresh adipose tissues before ADSC cryopreservation or isolated from cryopreserved fat tissues, showed unaltered capabilities of proliferation and differentiation after optimal cryopreservation protocols, which confirms the probability of ADSCs providing an important source for cell-based therapy and tissue engineering (**Fig. 4**). Further extensive studies in cryopreservation of adipose cells and tissues are expected to further benefit the applications of fat transplantation, including development of novel cryoprotection media (DMSO free, serum free, and even xeno free), more fundamental cryobiological studies of adipose cells and tissues, and optimization and standardization of the fat cryopreservation protocols for producing GMP products. Successful cryopreservation of adipose tissue and ADSCs can lead to a new era in fat grafting and ADSC-related tissue regeneration therapy in plastic surgery.

REFERENCES

1. Coleman SR. Structural fat grafts - the ideal filler? Clin Plast Surg 2001;28:111–9.
2. Wolter TP, von Heimburg D, Stoffels I, et al. Cryopreservation of mature human adipocytes - in vitro measurement of viability. Ann Plast Surg 2005;55: 408–13.
3. Raskin BI. Cryopreserved fat. In: Shiffman MA, editor. Autologous fat transfer: art, science, and clinical practice. New York: Springer; 2010. p. 305–11.
4. Butterwick KJ, Bevin AA, Iyer S. Fat transplantation using fresh versus frozen fat: a side-by-side two-hand comparison pilot study. Dermatol Surg 2006; 32:640–4.
5. Shoshani O, Ullmann Y, Shupak A, et al. The role of frozen storage in preserving adipose tissue obtained by suction-assisted lipectomy for repeated fat injection procedures. Dermatol Surg 2001;27:645–7.
6. MacRae JW, Tholpady SS, Ogle RC, et al. Ex vivo fat graft preservation - effects and implications of cryopreservation. Ann Plast Surg 2004;52:281–2.
7. Pu LL, Cui X, Fink FB, et al. Long-term preservation of adipose aspirates after conventional lipoplasty. Aesthet Surg J 2004;24:536–41.
8. Moscatello DK, Dougherty M, Narins RS, et al. Cryopreservation of human fat for soft tissue augmentation: viability requires use of cryoprotectant and controlled freezing and storage. Dermatol Surg 2005;31:1506–10.
9. Pu LL, Cui X, Fink BF, et al. Cryopreservation of adipose tissues: the role of trehalose. Aesthet Surg J 2005;25:126–31.
10. Atik B, Ozturk G, Erdogan E, et al. Comparison of techniques for long-term storage of fat grafts: an experimental study. Plast Reconstr Surg 2006;118: 1533–7.
11. Pu LL, Cui X, Li J, et al. The fate of cryopreserved adipose aspirates after in vivo transplantation. Aesthet Surg J 2006;26:653–61.
12. Pu LL, Cui XD, Fink BF, et al. Adipose aspirates as a source for human processed lipoaspirate cells after optimal cryopreservation. Plast Reconstr Surg 2006; 117:1845–50.
13. Cui XD, Gao DY, Fink BF, et al. Cryopreservation of human adipose tissues. Cryobiology 2007;55: 269–78.
14. Cui XD, Gao DY, Fink BF, et al. Cryopreservation of composite tissues and transplantation: preliminary studies. Cryobiology 2007;55:295–304.
15. Goh BC, Thirumala S, Kilroy G, et al. Cryopreservation characteristics of adipose-derived stem cells: maintenance of differentiation potential and viability. J Tissue Eng Regen Med 2007;1:322–4.
16. Gonda K, Shigeura T, Sato T, et al. Preserved proliferative capacity and multipotency of human adipose-derived stem cells after long-term cryopreservation. Plast Reconstr Surg 2008;121:401–10.
17. Oishi K, Noguchi H, Yukawa H, et al. Cryopreservation of mouse adipose tissue-derived stem/progenitor cells. Cell Transpl 2008;17:35–41.
18. Cui XD, Pu LL. The search for a useful method for the optimal cryopreservation of adipose aspirates: part I. In vitro study. Aesthet Surg J 2009;29:248–52.
19. De Rosa A, De Francesco F, Tirino V, et al. A new method for cryopreserving adipose-derived stem cells: an attractive and suitable large-scale and long-term cell banking technology. Tissue Eng Part C Methods 2009;15:659–67.
20. Mambelli LI, Santos EJ, Frazao PJ, et al. Characterization of equine adipose tissue-derived progenitor cells before and after cryopreservation. Tissue Eng Part C Methods 2009;15:87–94.
21. Pu LL. Cryopreservation of adipose tissue. Organogenesis 2009;5:138–42.
22. Cui XD, Pu LL. The search for a useful method for the optimal cryopreservation of adipose aspirates: part II. In vivo study. Aesthet Surg J 2010;30:451–6.
23. Pu LL, Coleman SR, Cui XD, et al. Cryopreservation of autologous fat grafts harvested with the Coleman technique. Ann Plast Surg 2010;64:333–7.
24. Son D, Oh J, Choi T, et al. Viability of fat cells over time after syringe suction lipectomy the effects of cryopreservation. Ann Plast Surg 2010;65:354–60.
25. Thirumala S, Gimble JM, Devireddy RV. Evaluation of methylcellulose and dimethyl sulfoxide as the cryoprotectants in a serum-free freezing media for cryopreservation of adipose-derived adult stem cells. Stem Cells Dev 2010;19:513–22.
26. Thirumala S, Wu XY, Gimble JM, et al. Evaluation of polyvinylpyrrolidone as a cryoprotectant for adipose tissue-derived adult stem cells. Tissue Eng Part C Methods 2010;16:783–92.
27. Li BW, Liao WC, Wu SH, et al. Cryopreservation of fat tissue and application in autologous fat graft: in vitro and in vivo study. Aesthet Plast Surg 2012; 36:714–22.
28. Miyamoto Y, Oishi K, Yukawa H, et al. Cryopreservation of human adipose tissue-derived stem/progenitor cells using the silk protein sericin. Cell Transpl 2012;21:617–22.
29. Wang WZ, Fang XH, Williams SJ, et al. The effect of lipoaspirates cryopreservation on adipose-derived stem cells. Aesthet Surg J 2013;33:1046–55.
30. Chaput B, Orio J, Garrido I, et al. A clinical scalable cryopreservation method of adipose tissue for reconstructive surgery assessed by stromal

vascular fraction and mice studies. Plast Reconstr Surg 2014;133:815–26.

31. Choudhery MS, Badowski M, Muise A, et al. Cryopreservation of whole adipose tissue for future use in regenerative medicine. J Surg Res 2014; 187:24–35.

32. Devireddy R. Cryopreservation of adipose tissue derived adult stem cells. J Tissue Eng Regen Med 2014;8:154.

33. Mazur P. Kinetics of water loss from cells at subzero temperatures and likelihood of intracellular freezing. J Gen Physiol 1963;47:347–69.

34. Mazur P. Cryobiology: the freezing of biological systems. Science 1970;168:939–49.

35. Diller KR. Quantitative low temperature optical microscopy of biological systems. J Microsc 1982; 126:9–28.

36. Gao DY, Benson CT, Liu C, et al. Development of a novel microperfusion chamber for determination of cell membrane transport properties. Biophys J 1996;71:443–50.

37. Chen HH, Purtteman JJ, Heimfeld S, et al. Development of a microfluidic device for determination of cell osmotic behavior and membrane transport properties. Cryobiology 2007;55:200–9.

38. Toner M, Cravalho EG, Karel M. Thermodynamics and kinetics of intracellular ice formation during freezing of biological cells. J Appl Phys 1990;67: 1582–93.

39. Karlsson JO, Cravalho EG, Toner M. A model of diffusion-limited ice growth inside biological cells during freezing. J Appl Phys 1994;75:4442–5.

40. Gao DY, Liu J, Liu C, et al. Prevention of osmotic injury to human spermatozoa during addition and removal of glycerol. Hum Reprod 1995;10:1109–22.

41. Karlsson JO, Toner M. Long-term storage of tissues by cryopreservation: critical issues. Biomaterials 1996;17:243–56.

42. Grewal N, Yacomotti L, Melkonyan V, et al. Freezing adipose tissue grafts may damage their ability to integrate into the host. Connect Tissue Res 2009; 50:14–28.

43. Gao D, Critser JK. Mechanisms of cryoinjury in living cells. ILAR J 2000;41:187–96.

44. Crowe JH, Crowe LM, Oliver AE, et al. The trehalose myth revisited: introduction to a symposium on stabilization of cells in the dry state. Cryobiology 2001;43:89–105.

45. Shu Z, Heimfeld S, Gao D. Hematopoietic SCT with cryopreserved grafts: adverse reactions after transplantation and cryoprotectant removal before infusion. Bone Marrow Transpl 2014;49:469–76.

46. Liu GP, Zhou H, Li YL, et al. Evaluation of the viability and osteogenic differentiation of cryopreserved human adipose-derived stem cells. Cryobiology 2008;57:18–24.

47. Davies OG, Smith AJ, Cooper PR, et al. The effects of cryopreservation on cells isolated from adipose, bone marrow and dental pulp tissues. Cryobiology 2014;69:342–7.

48. Germann A, Schulz JC, Kemp-Kamke B, et al. Standardized serum-free cryomedia maintain peripheral blood mononuclear cell viability, recovery, and antigen-specific T-cell response compared to fetal calf serum-based medium. Biopreserv Biobank 2011;9:229–36.

49. Schulz JC, Germann A, Kemp-Kamke B, et al. Towards a xeno-free and fully chemically defined cryopreservation medium for maintaining viability, recovery, and antigen-specific functionality of PBMC during long-term storage. J Immunol Methods 2012;382:24–31.

Fat Grafting in Facial Rejuvenation

Timothy J. Marten, MD*, Dino Elyassnia, MD

KEYWORDS

- Fat injections • Fat transfer • Autologous fat grafting • Microfat grafting • Facelift • Facial atrophy
- Stem cell facelift • Fat grafting complications

KEY POINTS

- Fat grafting areas of the face that have atrophied with age can produce a significant and sustained improvement in appearance and improved outcomes in facelift procedures.
- Fat grafting provides for volumetric rejuvenation, which is a new and different means to improve facial appearance, and a new dimension for plastic surgeons to work in.
- In addition, fat grafting may induce an improvement in facial tissue quality through an as-yet undefined stem cell effect.

THE AGING FACE AND THE NEED FOR FAT GRAFTING

Recognizing the changes that occur as the face ages and appreciating the underlying anatomic problems responsible for them is essential to properly advising patients and planning surgical procedures. In most patients, problems will fall into in 3 general categories:

1. Aging and breakdown of the skin surface
2. Tissue sagging, skin redundancy, and loss of youthful facial contour
3. Facial hollowing and atrophy

Skin care and skin resurfacing procedure address changes in the first category. Traditional lifts of the face, neck, forehead, and eyes address the second.[1–12] Fat grafting allows clinicians to treat atrophy, something they were previously unable to do, and is now acknowledged by plastic surgeons and other physicians engaged in treating the aging face as the most important advance in aesthetic surgery in several decades or more. Properly performed, the addition of fat to areas of the face that have atrophied because of age or disease can produce a significant and sustained improvement in appearance that is unobtainable by other means. All things being otherwise equal, simultaneous facelift and fat grafting produce a better result than either technique performed alone, and when a facelift is performed in conjunction with fat grafting both loss of contour and facial atrophy can be corrected, and optimal improvement can be obtained (**Fig. 1**).

VOLUMETRIC REJUVENATION, TISSUE INTEGRATION, AND STEM CELL EFFECT

Fat grafting provides volumetric rejuvenation; a new and different means by which to improve facial appearance, and a new dimension for plastic surgeons to work in. Unlike nonautologous injectables, fat integrates with facial tissues, becomes part of the face, and produces an arguably more natural-appearing, sustained, and long-lasting improvement. In addition, fat grafting may induce an improvement in facial tissue quality through an as-yet not clearly defined stem cell effect, and when performed with a facelift may constitute, for the first time, rejuvenation in the true sense of the word.

Marten Clinic of Plastic Surgery, San Francisco, CA 94108, USA
* Corresponding author.
E-mail address: info@martenclinic.com

Clin Plastic Surg 42 (2015) 219–252
http://dx.doi.org/10.1016/j.cps.2014.12.003

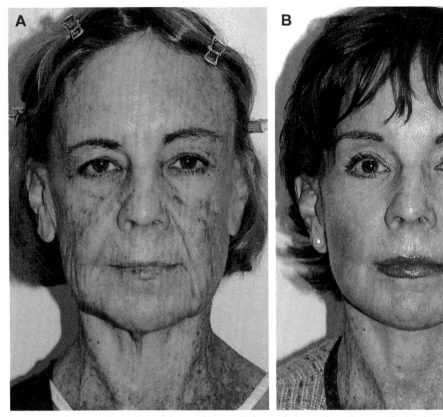

Fig. 1. Simultaneous facelift and fat grafting. All things being otherwise equal, simultaneous facelift and fat grafting produces a better result than either technique performed alone. (*A*) Patient with tissue ptosis and redundancy, and marked facial atrophy. (*B*) Same patient seen 14 months after high superficial muscular aponeurotic system (SMAS) facelift, neck lift, closed forehead lift, upper and lower blepharoplasties, and panfacial fat grafting. (note: patient has had hyaluronic acid filler placed in lips). (*Courtesy of* Marten Clinic of Plastic Surgery. All surgical procedures performed by Timothy J. Marten, MD, FACS, San Francisco, CA.)

DRAWBACKS OF FAT GRAFTING

Performing fat grafting in conjunction with a facelift has certain disadvantages, including the learning curve associated with any new procedure, an increase in operating room time, increased post operative edema, a longer period of recovery, and uncertainty of graft take. Certain patient misconceptions misconceptions will also encountered and will have to including misguided beliefs that injected fat can migrate or fall, or that fat grafting makes the face look fat.

WHY NOT JUST GRAFT FAT?

Age-related loss of facial fat rarely exists as an isolated event and thus patients troubled by it are rarely logically or appropriately treated by fat grafting alone. Isolated fat grafting is also of questionable benefit to patients troubled by significant facial sagging and skin redundancy. Although aggressive filling of the sagging face with fat can produce improved contour and a smoother-appearing skin surface, it generally results in an unusually large, overfilled face that appears both unnatural and unfeminine. Such an overfilled face is difficult to correct in an attractive manner at a later date, and it is both more logical and practical to perform fat grafting in conjunction with formal surgical lifts if needed, or at some time after ptotic tissue has been repositioned and redundant tissue has been removed. Our contemporary concept for facial rejuvenation can thus be summarized as one in which surgical lifts are used to reposition sagging facial tissues and reduce the size of the facial skin envelope, and fat grafting is then used synergistically, but more appropriately and effectively, to restore areas that are truly volume depleted.

WHERE SHOULD THE FAT BE INJECTED PLACED?

Areas in need of treatment vary from patient to patient, and planning a fat grafting procedure requires looking at the face in a different way; more as a sculptor and less as a tailor as surgeons have done in the past. Any area successfully treatable with nonautologous injectable fillers is potentially treatable with fat grafting, including, but not limited to, the temples, forehead, brow, glabella, radix, upper orbit (upper eyelid), lower orbit (lower eyelid), cheeks, tear trough, midface, lips, perioral, stomal angles, nasolabial crease, geniomandibular groove (GMG), jawline, chin crease, submental crease, and chin areas, and personal experience with fillers is a useful point of reference for planning fat additions to the face. In time, and after engaging thoughtfully in study of the aging face, surgeons will gain a deeper appreciation of facial atrophy and an increasing desire to correct it. **Fig. 2** shows a patient before and after facelift and fat grafting, and the areas where fat was placed.

SEQUENCING FAT GRAFTING WITH OTHER PROCEDURES

Although there is no consensus on when fat grafting is best performed during facelift surgery, as a practical matter it is most expedient to inject fat at the beginning of the procedure, before the facelift has been performed. The reasons for this include that it is easier to harvest the fat at the beginning of the procedure before the face has been prepped or draped and when the patient is typically in a deeper plane of anesthesia. In the beginning of the procedure the tissue planes of the face have also not been opened, the face is not swollen, and preoperatively made pen marks and facial landmarks are easier to identify. In addition, surgical principles suggest that it is best to limit the time the graft is out of the body. However, perhaps the most important reason to do the fat grafting first is that surgeons are more technically and artistically energetic in the morning, and do a better job than if the procedure is performed at the end of a long facelift procedure.

LOGISTICS OF SIMULTANEOUS FACELIFT AND FAT GRAFTING

Fat grafting is often mistakenly thought to be a simple procedure that can be performed in a few minutes, but this is rarely the case, and such an attitude leads to frustration, disruption of workflow, and poor outcomes. For the procedure to be successful, fat must be harvested in a specific

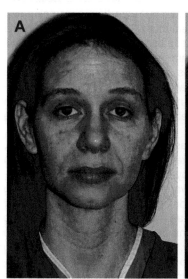
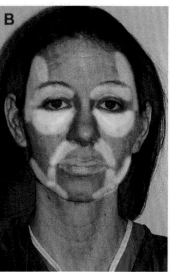
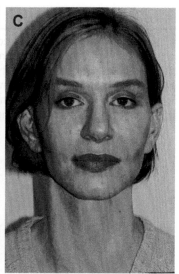

Fig. 2. ABC Patient Before and After Simultaneous Facelift and Fat Injections. (*A*) A 47 year old patient before procedure. She has had no prior surgery. (*B*) Shaded areas showing were fat was placed. 1 cc was placed in each upper orbit, 3 cc was placed in each temple, 1 cc was placed in each tear trough, 3 cc was placed in each infra-orbital area, 2 cc was placed in each cheek, 2 cc was placed in each nasolabial crease, 1 cc was placed in each stomal angle, 1 cc was placed in each geniomandibular groove, 3 cc placed along each jawline, and 1 cc was placed in each lip. (*C*) Same patient 1 year and 1 month after high SMAS facelift, neck lift, upper blepharoplasty (levator re-insertion), lower blepharoplasty, upper lip lift, and 38 cc of fat injections. (*Courtesy of* Marten Clinic of Plastic Surgery. All surgical procedures performed by Timothy J. Marten, MD, FACS, San Francisco, CA.)

time-consuming manner and it must then be processed and infiltrated in a technically demanding and time-consuming process. Fat grafting is also an artistically demanding activity that requires a considerable amount of the surgeon's creative energy. When anything other than a few small areas of the face are being treated the procedure can easily encompass an hour or more, something that can overburden a surgical team already engaged in a long and demanding facelift operation consisting of multiple procedures. Time must therefore be planned and allocated accordingly.

FAT INJECTION TECHNIQUE

The basic technique for fat grafting has been described previously,[1] and the principles set forth by Coleman[13] are observed when fat grafting is performed.

Needed Equipment

Special instruments are required for fat harvest and injection (**Fig. 3**), in addition to a few other pieces of equipment used to process and organize the fat (www.tulipmedical.com, www.mentorwwllc.com). Other than for intradermal injections, sharp hypodermic needles should not be used to inject fat because fat embolization and serious related problems, including tissue infarction and visual impairment and blindness, can occur.

Choosing a Fat Harvest Site

At present there is no scientific consensus as to what is the best site to harvest fat from for fat grafting procedures. Harvest sites are typically chosen and marked in a manner to improve the patient's figure, although the ideal locations are arguably fat collections resistant to diet and exercise. For

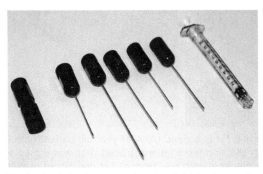

Fig. 3. Fat injection cannulas. Special blunt cannulas are required to safely perform fat grafting and poor outcomes are likely if sharp hypodermic needles are used. Sharp needle injection also poses a risk of fat embolization and related problems.

women this is typically the hip, outer thigh, or abdomen, and for men the love-handle and spare-tire areas. In thin patients, small harvests from multiple areas are required, and additional time must be allotted for this in the procedure. It is prudent for the sites marked for harvest to be photographed preoperatively to document what was agreed on, and to avoid any disagreement over the preoperative condition of fat harvest sites after surgery.

Preoperative Marking of the Face

Fat grafting cannot be performed casually, and deficient areas and key landmarks must be marked preoperatively with the patient in an upright position. Marking requires concentration and focus, and is best performed in an area that is private and free from distractions. Creating a proposed plan on a full-page laser print of a photograph of the patient's face is helpful in organizing the treatment plan, and facilitates confirming with the patient the areas that will be treated. If patients wish, marks can be made while they hold a hand mirror. Once markings are complete, a new series of photographs are taken and printed up for use during the procedure. These photographs typically provide the best information to the surgeon during surgery.

Anesthesia

Well-performed facelifts are time consuming and technically demanding undertakings, and the addition of fat grafting to the procedure strains the patience and composure of most surgeons. As such, it is highly recommended that the services of an anesthesiologist or competent certified registered nurse anesthetists be enlisted when combined facelift and fat grafting procedures are performed.

Except in cases in which it is contraindicated, our facelifts are performed under deep sedation administered by an anesthesiologist using a laryngeal mask airway. This strategy allows patients to be heavily sedated while maintaining control of their airways, and the patients need not receive muscle relaxants and can be allowed to breathe spontaneously. Heavily sedated patients are also much easier to harvest fat from and comprehensively treat, especially when harvest needs to be made from multiple sites.

Harvesting Fat

Although the primary goal of fat harvest is to obtain the best tissue for the fat grafting procedure, fat harvesting should be thought of as an opportunity to improve the patient's figure, and as such harvest must be undertaken in a thoughtful and artistic manner and generally in a bilateral and symmetric fashion.

Thin patients should be examined at the time of their consultation because patients with limited fat stores often present significant challenges, and extra time and effort are required to obtain fat from them. Anesthesia and operating room times, and the surgeon's fee, must be calculated accordingly.

The abdomen is often cited as the best and most convenient site for fat harvest but when comprehensive treatment of the face is planned (or when the dorsum of the hands are being simultaneously treated), the amount of fat needed cannot always be readily obtained from the abdominal area alone. The abdomen also typically has thinner, less forgiving skin than the hip, waist, and outer thigh (especially in aged patients having facelifts), and is readily open to detailed inspection by the patient after the procedure. As such, it can be problematic as a sole donor site in many cases if more than a small amount of fat is needed. In contrast, the hip, waist, and outer thigh taken together typically provide more volume, are less subject to surface irregularities caused by poor skin contraction, and fat harvested from these areas generally provides more overall improvement in the patient's silhouette, and are therefore the primary harvest sites of choice in our practice.

An estimate should be made as to the amount of fat that will be used and thus the amount that needs to be harvested before fat harvest is undertaken. Smaller fat grafting procedures generally require 15 to 30 mL, intermediate procedures 30 to 50 mL, and comprehensive procedures can encompass the placement of 50 to 100 mL (occasionally more) and harvest must be made accordingly. In estimating the amount that needs to be harvested, a helpful guideline is that after centrifugation approximately 50% of what was harvested will on average be available as usable processed fat. If the clinician wishes to perform the fat grafting procedure predominantly with stem cell–rich fat (the bottom 2 mL of fat in the centrifuged 10-mL syringe, consisting of high-density adipocytes) only 20% of what is harvested fat will be available for injection and the total amount harvested must be adjusted accordingly.

As in the case of formal liposuction, the patient's torso must be marked preoperatively while the patient is standing if optimal contours are to be created and if irregularities are to be avoided at the harvest sites. Once markings are complete, marked areas should be photographed and the photographs printed for use during the harvesting part of the procedure.

Fat is harvested after anesthesia is initiated but before prep and drape of the face. A complete prep of the torso is not necessary and in all but unusual cases a limited prep of the marked area is made and a sterile field is established. If fat is to be harvested from the hip or lateral thigh, the patient is turned into a semilateral decubitus position; prep, drape, and harvest performed; and the patient then turned to the opposite side, where a similar procedure is performed. If the patient is positioned carefully, this position can be used to simultaneously harvest fat from multiple sites, including the hip, waist, flank, upper buttocks, outer and inner thigh, and knees (**Fig. 4**). With practice, a well-organized operating room team can complete this process expeditiously without undue delay of the overall procedure.

Areas from which fat is to be harvested are infiltrated with a dilute 0.1% lidocaine with 1:1,000,000 epinephrine solution using a multi-holed infiltration cannula (**Fig. 5**), and an adequate time allowed for a proper anesthetic and hemostatic effect. Approximately 1 mL of this solution is injected for every 3 mL of anticipated fat removal. It is not necessary or desirable to infiltrate tumescent fashion because overwetting the tissue results in an overdilute harvest and more time spent in the harvesting process. Local anesthetic should be injected even if general anesthesia is used to limit stimulation of the patient and the overall amount of general anesthetic used.

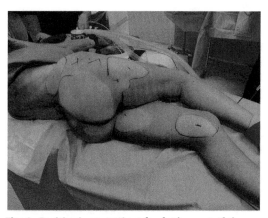

Fig. 4. Positioning a patient for fat harvest. If the patient is carefully positioned in a semilateral decubitus position, fat can simultaneously be harvested from multiple sites, including the hip waist, flank, inner knee, outer and inner thighs, buttocks, and inner knee. Obtaining fat from multiple sites is particularly important in thin patients with minimal fat stores or when multiple-site fat grafting is being performed. Following harvest from one side the patient is turned to the other, where a similar harvest is performed.

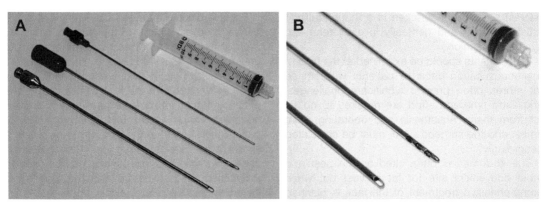

Fig. 5. Fat harvesting instruments. (*A*) Specially designed harvesting cannulas ranging in size from 2.1 to 2.4 mm are attached to 10-mL Luer lock syringes and are used to extract fat from donor sites using gentle syringe suction. Fat harvested with these cannulas easily passes through injection cannulas as small as 0.7 mm. Shown from top down: (1) 10-mL Luer lock syringe, (2) 1.6-mm Coleman local anesthetic infiltration cannula, (3) 2.4-mm Tulip Tri-port harvesting cannula, and (4) Coleman harvesting cannula. (*B*) Close-up of instrument tips. Shown from top down: (1) 10-mL Luer lock syringe, (2) Coleman infiltration cannula, (3) Tulip harvesting cannula, and (4) Coleman harvesting cannula.

Fat is harvested with a special harvesting cannula (see **Fig. 5**) ranging in size from 2.1 to 2.4 mm, and 15 to 25 cm long, attached to a 10-mL syringe using gently applied syringe suction to minimize vacuum barotrauma to the tissue. Sharp hypodermic needles should not be used. In general, and as mentioned previously, at least twice as much fat is harvested as is anticipated will be used to ensure that an adequate supply of processed fat will be available for use on the face.

Once fat harvest is complete, the stab incision used to obtain the fat is closed with a simple interrupted suture of 6-0 nylon. The harvest site is then washed free of prep solution and the sutured site dressed with a TegaDerm™ dressing.

Processing Harvested Fat

Harvested fat is generally not uniform in character and concentration as extracted and some type of processing is necessary to obtain uniform material for injection. Although fat can be separated from blood and local anesthetic using a tea strainer–type sieve or rolling it on Telfa™ gauze, most of the stem cells, growth factors, and chemical cellular messengers are likely to be lost when this is done. Centrifugation conversely allows separation of the oil (ruptured fat cells) and water (blood and local anesthetic) fractions from the fat cells while simultaneously concentrating these other potentially important components, and has been our favored method of fat processing for almost 2 decades.

Before centrifugation is commenced, a sterile disposable plastic cap is placed on the end of the syringe to keep its contents inside it, and the syringe plunger removed from the syringe barrel. Capped syringe barrels containing unprocessed fat are then loaded into the centrifuge in a balanced fashion and spun for 1 to 3 minutes at 1000 revolutions per minute (RPM). Many centrifuges available for this purpose have variable speed adjustments and rotors that can be sterilized so that the syringes containing the fat remain sterile and can be handled by the scrubbed surgical team. Others centrifuges have sterilizable tubes that fit into the rotor for this purpose (**Fig. 6**).

The typical spin speeds of approximately 3500 RPM used by most single-speed desktop centrifuges sold for fat processing are said to not cause injury to fat, or compromise its take.

Once centrifuged, syringe barrels containing spun fat are removed and centrifuged fat is seen to contain an upper oil (ruptured fat cells), central fat, and lower water (blood, lidocaine) components (**Fig. 7**).

The often blood-tinged water (local anesthetic) component is discarded by simply removing the syringe tip cap and allowing it to run out. The oil fraction is then poured off from the top of the syringe. Telfa™ sponges can also be placed inside the syringe barrel to wick up the small amount of residual oil present after most of it has been poured off (cotton sponges should not be used because fat would be contaminated with microscopic inflammatory fibers). A laboratory test tube–type rack to hold and organize

A

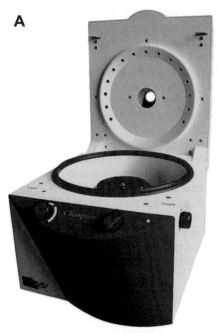

B

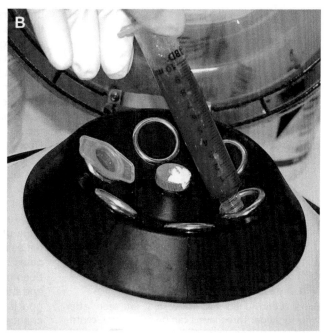

Fig. 6. Centrifuging fat. Harvested fat is generally not uniform in character as extracted from donor sites because each syringe contains a variable amount of fat, blood, local anesthetic, and ruptured fat cells (oil), and some type of processing is necessary to obtain uniform material for injection. Centrifugation allows separation of the oil and water fractions from the fat cells and concentrates high-density adipocytes (stem cells). (*A*) Small portable countertop centrifuge (www.tulipmedical.com). (*B*) Close-up view of centrifuge rotor being loaded with unprocessed fat in 10-mL syringes. Note that the syringe tip has been sealed with a disposable plastic cap. The removable and sterilizable metal sleeves shown fit into the rotor to keep syringe barrels containing fat sterile and allow them to be handled on the sterile field after spinning. Some centrifuges are designed to allow the entire rotor to be sterilized. (*Courtesy of* Tulip Medical, San Diego, CA; with permission.)

the syringes containing fat greatly facilitates fat processing activities (**Fig. 8**).

Injecting Fat

After centrifugation and the separation and discarding of the resulting oil and water components has been accomplished, the resultant fat is transferred into 1-mL Luer lock syringes using a transfer coupling (**Fig. 9**), because proper infiltration of fat requires injection in very small amounts that cannot reliably be made with 10-mL, 5-mL, or even 3-mL syringes. The bottom 2 mL of fat in the syringe containing the highest concentrations of high-density adipocytes (or adipose-derived regenerative cells) are segregated and are used preferentially in the procedure and for critical areas (orbits, lips, and tear trough). If an adequate over-harvest is made, enough high-density fat will be obtained for the entire facial fat grafting procedure.

Nerve blocks are then performed with 0.25% bupivacaine with epinephrine 1:200,000 local anesthetic solution. It is typically not necessary to directly infiltrate areas to be treated with local anesthetic in patients having facelifts if nerve

blocks are properly performed and adequate sedation has been administered.

Once nerve blocks have been administered, 0.7-mm, 0.9-mm, and 1.2-mm (22-gauge to 18-gauge) cannulas are used to infiltrate fat into the face through small stab incisions made in the facial skin with an 11-blade scalpel or a 20-gauge needle. These incisions are so small that they do not require suturing on completion of the procedure.

Infiltration is made in multiple passes, injecting on both the in and out strokes in planes appropriate for the area being treated, usually from 2 separate injection sites, and feathering into adjacent areas. Injecting from 2 separate injection sites allows crisscrossing of cannula passes during graft placement, provides smoother fat infiltration, and helps avert a row-of-corn effect that may result if injection is made from only 1 site.

How much should be injected?

Deciding how much fat needs to be injected at a given site requires empirical information and the surgeon cannot simply rely on what is seen in the

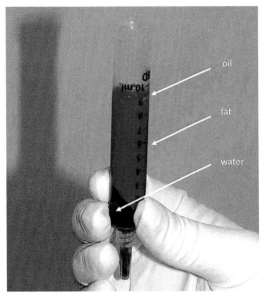

Fig. 7. Centrifuged fat. Harvested fat seen after centrifugation. Three layers can be seen in the centrifuged material: an upper oil layer (ruptured fat cells), a middle layer of intact fat cells, and a bottom layer of blood and local anesthetic. Unlike straining of fat through a sieve, centrifugation may allow separation of the oil and water fractions from the fat cells with minimal loss of stem cells, growth factors, and cellular messengers.

operating room. In most cases the amount needed exceeds what intuition and direct observation suggest and it is best decided preoperatively based on the degree of deficiency seen in the

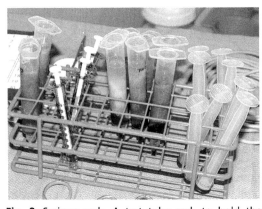

Fig. 8. Syringe rack. A test tube rack to hold the syringes containing fat greatly facilitates fat processing activities. On the left are syringes containing unprocessed fat. In the center, syringes containing centrifuged fat can be seen. The rack also conveniently holds 1-mL syringes, syringe components, and other equipment used in the fat grafting procedure.

preoperative photographs. As a practical matter, there is an empirical range and a small, medium, and large treatment within that range applicable to each site. For small problems, a volume at the low end of the empirical range is used. For medium-sized problems, a volume in the midrange is chosen. For large problems, an injection volume at the high end of the range is used.

How Is the fat injected?

As the cannula is advanced, tissue resistance is felt for, and if resistance is felt a small injection is made. Approximately 0.5 mL or less should be injected per pass, which corresponds with 20 to 40 back-and-forth passes or more for each 1-mL syringe of processed fat. If tissue resistance is not felt as the injection cannula is advanced, this indicates that a pass and injection has likely already been made in that area, so injection is not made and the cannula is directed to another area. The goal is to inject the fat in a way that optimizes its chances of developing a blood supply and surviving, and the mental model should be one of scattering tiny particles of fat into the recipient site in multiple crisscrossing fine trails in such a way that each particle sits in its own compartment and has maximal surface contact with perfused tissue. If fat is injected in a bolus, fat cells will be clumped together and only those on the periphery of the injected area will have tissue contact and be likely survive. Most of the more centrally situated fat particles will only have contact with each other, will be less likely to survive, and can lead to the formation of oil cysts. Put in more practical terms, the procedure should be thought of as analogous to spray painting and not caulking.

Advancement and withdrawal of the injection cannula is typically made slowly by the beginning injector, but, as familiarity with the technique is acquired, the movements can and should be made faster. Ultimately, all other things being equal, faster movements are desirable in that, if the injection cannula is constantly in motion, intravascular injection is less likely, and the likelihood that an accidental bolus injection into one area will be made is reduced. Rapid back-and-forth movements also ensure the smoothest and most uniform infiltration of fat.

How the syringe is held is also important in avoiding overinjection and controlling the volume injected with each pass. If the syringe is held in the manner that would traditionally be used to give an injection, with the thumb on the end of the syringe plunger, it is easy to inject too much fat if tissue resistance changes or injection cannula resistance suddenly decreases. More control can generally be maintained, and overinjection more

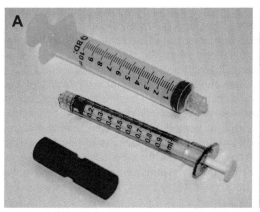
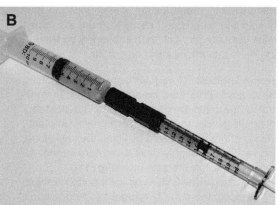

Fig. 9. Transferring centrifuged fat to 1-mL syringes. Fat is transferred from 10-mL Luer lock syringes into 1-mL Luer lock syringes after centrifugation and the oil and water fractions have been discarded using a transfer coupling. Proper injection in the small quantities that are needed in the face cannot be made with larger syringes. (*A*) A 10-mL Luer lock syringe, 1 mL Luer lock syringe, and Luer-to-Luer transfer coupling. (*B*) Transfer coupling in use.

easily avoided, if the syringe is held with the end of the plunger in the palm of the hand (**Fig. 10**). Held in this manner, a slight closing of the hand results in a small amount of fat only being expressed from the cannula, and overinjection of any area can more readily be avoided.

Although cannula obstruction is uncommon if fat is harvested and processed as previously described, if a cannula becomes blocked additional injection pressure should not be applied because this is the most common cause of a sudden and unintentional bolus injection. It is better in

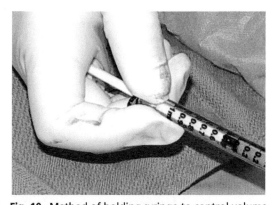

Fig. 10. Method of holding syringe to control volume expressed during injection. If the syringe is held in the way that would traditionally be used to give an injection it is easy to inject too much fat if tissue or injection cannula resistance suddenly decreases. More control can be maintained, and overinjection better avoided, if the syringe is held with the end of the plunger in the palm of the hand. Held in this manner, a slight closing of the hand results in only a small amount of fat being expressed.

such circumstances simply to withdraw the blocked cannula, pass it to the surgical assistant, and continue with a different one. The assistant can then clear the obstruction while the surgeon continues to work with the second cannula. The cause of the obstruction is typically a particle of fat at the interface of the cannula and the cannula hub, which is most easily cleared by removing the cannula from the syringe and extracting it from inside the hub with a fine forceps.

How deep should the fat be grafted and in what layers should fat be placed?

Fat grafts need to be placed in different planes depending on the areas being treated and the problem that is present. In many areas where there are multiple tissue layers to inject in and the overlying skin is thick, injection can be made comprehensively at the treated site from periosteum to the subdermal layer. These areas typically include the GMG, piriform, midface, cheek, and the chin. In other areas, fat grafts must be placed more specifically because of the anatomic characteristics and constraints of the treated sites if optimal results are to be obtained and irregularities are to be avoided. These areas include the temples (which often must be injected subcutaneously); the upper orbit, lower orbit, and tear trough, which should be injected in a preperiosteal/sub–orbicularis oculi plane; the lips, which should be injected predominantly in a submucosal plane; and the jawline, which should be injected in a preperiosteal/submasseteric plane. The easiest areas for beginning injectors to treat are the sites in the first category. In addition, in the beginning it is wise to stay deep and place most of the graft in a predominantly preperiosteal plane. Once familiarity with the technique has been obtained, areas in the last category can then cautiously be treated and more superficial injections made.

Geniomandibular ("pre-jowl") groove Fat grafting the prejowl/GMG area creates a strong, uninterrupted aesthetic line from chin to the posterior mandible (similar to the effect of a prejowl implant), which cannot be achieved by lifting the jowl alone, and results in a highly desirable improvement on both the male and female face (**Fig. 11**).

Fat grafting of the GMG is typically performed with a 4 cm long, 0.7-mm (22-gauge) injection cannula from injection sites over the mandibular border and on the perioral area (**Fig. 12**) and fat is placed in all tissue layers between the periosteum and skin.

From 1 to 3 mL of fat are typically placed on each side in the prejowl/GMG area, depending on the size of the depression present, but occasionally more is indicated. Fat grafting the GMG is less difficult than other areas and is a good area for beginners to start on.

Cheek Fat grafting the check can enhance facial shape and proportion and produce the kind of improvements obtained when Terino malar, Binder submalar, and combined malar-submalar shell-style cheek implants are placed (**Fig. 13**). In some cases it can be argued that fat grafting of the cheek produces a softer, better integrated, and more natural and feminine-appearing improvement in malar contour than implant placement (discussed later).

Fat grafting of the cheek is typically performed with a 5 cm long, 0.7-mm (22-gauge) injection cannula from injection sites situated on the midcheek and perioral areas (**Fig. 14**) and fat is placed in all tissue layers between the periosteum and skin.

Between 3 and 7 mL of fat are typically placed on each side in the cheek area, depending on the degree of atrophy present, but occasionally more is indicated. Often an asymmetrical placement and/or different amounts of fat are required on the right and left sides because of the presence of preexisting malar asymmetry. The cheek is also a good area for beginning injectors to treat.

Chin Fat grafting the chin can correct age-associated loss of chin volume, loss of chin projection, and loss of vertical chin height, and in some cases can rival the kind of improvements obtained when small chin implants are placed (**Fig. 15**).

Fat grafting of the chin can also correct an atrophic and feeble appearance that occurs as the chin shrinks with age by broadening and strengthening it (**Fig. 16**), and filling in the labiomental and submental creases when indicated. Typically, treatment of the chin must be undertaken in conjunction with the GMG, and the 2 areas overlap each other in most cases.

Fat grafting of the chin is typically performed with a 4 cm long, 0.7-mm (22-gauge) cannula from injection sites slightly lateral to the area being treated. Occasionally a third incision is used near the midline of the lower lip (**Fig. 17**). Fat is typically placed in all tissue layers from periosteum and skin.

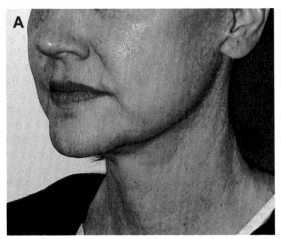 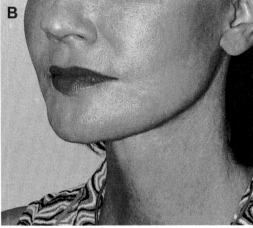

Fig. 11. Treatment of the GMG with fat grafting. (*A*) Patient with deep GMG seen preoperatively. The chin appears narrow and pointed, and there is poor continuity between the chin and jawline. (*B*) Same patient seen after facelift and injection of fat to fill the GMG (prejowl sulcus) area. A chin implant was not placed. The chin appears broader and more aesthetically integrated with the jawline. Fat was also used to strengthen the posterior jawline and lower the mandibular angle, and to fill the lips, nasolabial crease, cheeks, and infraorbital areas. (*Courtesy of* Marten Clinic of Plastic Surgery. All surgical procedures performed by Timothy J. Marten, MD, FACS, San Francisco, CA.)

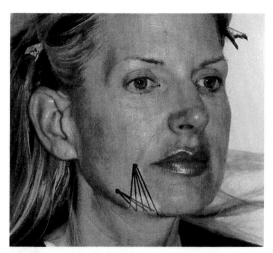

Fig. 12. Incision sites and plan for injecting fat into the prejowl/GMG areas. Fat grafting of the prejowl/GMG is performed with a 4-cm, 0.7-mm (22-gauge) cannula and fat is placed in all tissue layers between the periosteum and skin. Typically 1 to 3 mL of fat are placed on each side. Level of difficulty: beginner.

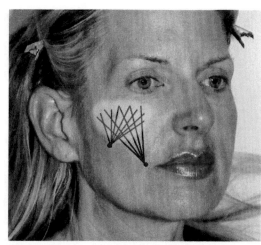

Fig. 14. Incision sites and plan for injecting fat into the cheek area. Fat grafting of the cheeks is typically performed with a 5-cm, 0.7-mm (22-gauge) cannula and fat is placed in all tissue layers between the periosteum and skin. Typically 3 to 7 mL of fat are placed in each cheek. Level of difficulty: beginner.

Between 1 and 3 mL of fat are typically placed in each side of the chin, depending on its size and shape and degree of atrophy, but occasionally more is indicated. Fat grafting the chin is intermediate in difficulty.

Fat grafts to the chin are best used for small augmentations only and cannot substitute for chin implants in all cases. If large changes in chin projection are attempted (and more than 3 mL of fat per side are used) a globular and less sculptural appearance is usually obtained, and patients in need of larger increases in chin projection are better treated with chin implants.

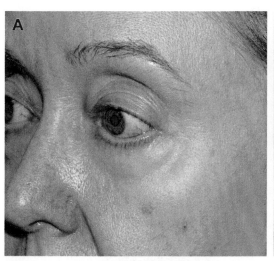

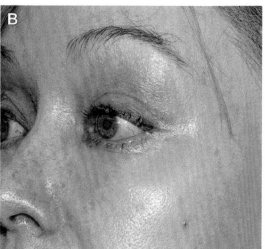

Fig. 13. Enhancing the cheeks with fat. As the cheek atrophies the lower eyelid fat bags become more exposed and prominent (pseudoherniation). Removing lower eyelid fat in such circumstances would create a hollow and elderly appearance and a low lid-cheek junction. (*A*) Patient with atrophic cheek and pseudoherniation of lower eyelid fat. The lower lid fat is exposed and appears ostensibly as a bag. (*B*) Same patient seen after fat grafting of the cheeks but no blepharoplasty. Protruding lower eyelid fat has been disguised by building up the cheek to produce a more youthful, fit, and attractive appearance than removing lower lid fat would have (note: the upper orbit has been replenished with fat grafts as well). (*Courtesy of* Marten Clinic of Plastic Surgery. All surgical procedures performed by Timothy J. Marten, MD, FACS, San Francisco, CA.)

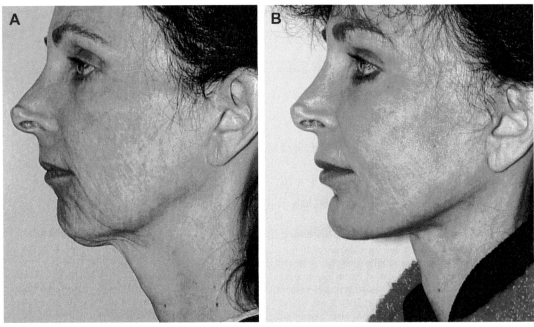

Fig. 15. Using fat grafting to project the chin. (*A*) Patient with underprojected chin seen before secondary facelift and fat grafting. The patient had previously had a chin implant inserted and removed by an unknown surgeon. (*B*) Same patient seen after secondary facelift with fat grafting of the chin. A chin implant was not placed. Injection of the chin with fat can enhance a patient's profile and, as shown, approach the kind of improvements obtained when small chin implants are placed (fat was also placed in the upper and lower orbits, cheeks, lips, and jawline areas). (*Courtesy of* Marten Clinic of Plastic Surgery. All surgical procedures performed by Timothy J. Marten, MD, FACS, San Francisco, CA.)

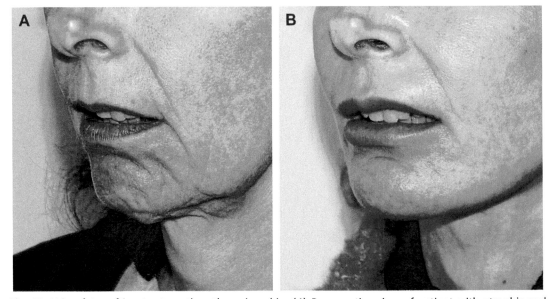

Fig. 16. Using fat grafting to strengthen the aging chin. (*A*) Preoperative view of patient with atrophic and feeble-appearing deflated chin. (*B*) Same patient seen after secondary facelift and fat grafting of the chin, GMG (prejowl sulcus), and jawline areas. A chin implant was not placed. The atrophic and feeble appearance was corrected with fat grafting by broadening and strengthening the chin. Treatment of the chin along with the GMG and jawline areas strengthens the lower facial contour. (*Courtesy of* Marten Clinic of Plastic Surgery. All surgical procedures performed by Timothy J. Marten, MD, FACS, San Francisco, CA.)

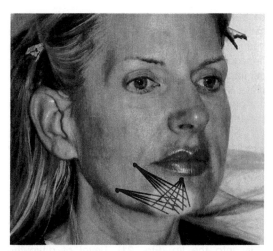

Fig. 17. Incision sites and plan for injecting fat into the chin. Fat grafting of the chin is typically performed with a 4-cm, 0.7-mm (22-gauge) cannula and fat is placed in all tissue layers between the periosteum and skin. Typically 1 to 3 mL of fat are placed in each side of the chin. Level of difficulty: intermediate.

Nasolabial injection Fat is an excellent adjunct in the treatment of the nasolabial fold in patients having facelifts (**Fig. 18**).

How and where fat is injected when treating the nasolabial fold depends on the type of problem. Injections should be made more superficially and predominantly subcutaneously if the nasolabial crease is being treated. Injections should be placed more deeply and predominantly over the piriform in the upper nasolabial area for age-associated maxillary recession. In many patients it is advantageous for both areas to be injected.

A 4 cm long, 0.7-mm (22-gauge) cannula is typically used and 1 to 3 mL of fat are placed in the nasolabial crease/fold area on each side, depending on the size of the problem. Fat grafting the nasolabial area is intermediate in difficulty (**Fig. 19**).

Overfilling the nasolabial area can produce changes in the posture of the patient's mouth and the shape of the smile, and can result in a change in the patient's appearance. For these reasons it is important for the surgeon to set reasonable goals and to limit the amount of fat placed to a reasonable amount.

It is also the case that treatment of the nasolabial crease is significantly enhanced when cheek atrophy is concomitantly addressed. In essence, filling the deflated cheek helps "lift" the nasolabial fold. In addition, a nasolabial crease appears less objectionable and more natural when the nasolabial fold overlying it is integrated and incorporated into the cheek mass.

Lips Treating the lips with fat has distinct advantages and disadvantages but, if the procedure is successful and graft take is good, patients are spared the inconvenience, discomfort, and expense of having to undergo repeated filler treatments and the many problems associated with lip implants and a variety of other types of lip grafts. Fat grafting also produces a soft, natural-appearing improvement, and usually an undercorrection that is arguably appropriate and desirable for typical patients having facelifts who are in need of some improvement in their mouths (**Fig. 20**).

Fat grafting the lips has the disadvantage that it usually produces a large amount of swelling that is slow to resolve, and that the take of the graft varies from patient to patient. Patients seeking a quick recovery, a specific lip size or shape, or nuanced changes are not optimal candidates for the procedure. Patients should also be advised that when using fat it is generally not possible to create the

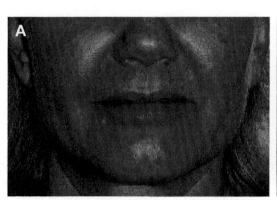
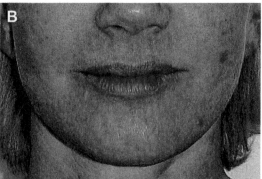

Fig. 18. Combined lifting and filling of the nasolabial fold. (*A*) Patient with midface ptosis and heavy nasolabial fold. (*B*) Same patient seen after high SMAS facelift and fat grafting of the nasolabial creases. A combined lifting and filling provides a better improvement than either procedure performed alone. (*Courtesy of* Marten Clinic of Plastic Surgery. All surgical procedures performed by Timothy J. Marten, MD, FACS, San Francisco, CA.)

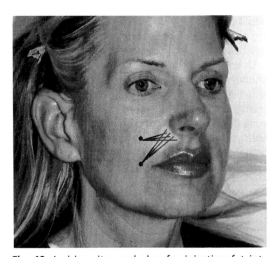

Fig. 19. Incision sites and plan for injecting fat into the piriform and nasolabial crease area. Fat grafting of the piriform and nasolabial crease is typically performed with a 4-cm, 0.7-mm (22-gauge) cannula. Fat is placed subcutaneously and superficially if treatment of the nasolabial skin crease is being made. Fat is placed preperiosteally if improvement in age-associated maxillary recession is indicated and desired. Fat is placed in all tissue layers between the periosteum and skin if both problems are present and are being treated. Typically 1 to 3 mL of fat are placed on each side. Level of difficulty: intermediate.

protrudes into the surgical field). The lips are typically treated after all other areas of the face have been fat grafted but before the facelift is begun because it requires the surgeon to insert his or her fingers inside the mouth. After injection is complete, the surgeon can remove and replace his or her outer gloves and the anterior face and mouth can then be reprepped.

A 5 cm long, 0.7-mm (22-gauge) cannula is used to infiltrate fat into the lips, but a slightly larger diameter cannula may be easier for beginning injectors because it is harder to accidentally perforate the mucosa or vermillion when a larger instrument is used. Injection is made from access incisions at each stomal angle, and fat is generally infiltrated superficially and submucosally into the lip (**Fig. 21**). Level of difficulty: intermediate.

The first few passes of the cannula are typically used to place fat directly under the vermillion-cutaneous junction, then under the red roll, and then under the white roll. Fat is then infiltrated submucosally beneath the wet and dry lip vermillion. If more lip protrusion is desired, additional fat is placed submucosally beneath the dry vermillion. If more vertical lip show is desired, more fat can be placed submucosally along the wet-dry junction of the vermillion on the inner aspect of the lip. A total of 1 to 1.5 mL (upper) to 1.5 to 2 mL (lower) is usually placed in each side of each lip for a total of 2 to 3 mL in the upper lip and 3 to 4 mL in the lower lip. Fat grafting the lips is intermediate in difficulty.

highly stylized cover-girl lip appearance seen in fashion magazines. These appearances are best obtained using nonautologous fillers.

When the surgical plan includes fat grafting of the lips, the prep of the face should include the upper and lower gingivobuccal sulci, the labial surface of the anterior teeth, and the tongue (if it

Perioral area and pucker lines Traditional resurfacing by peel, laser, or dermabrasion typically provides an incomplete solution for patients with

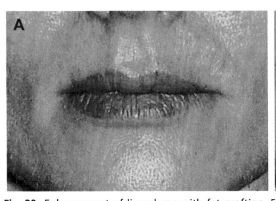
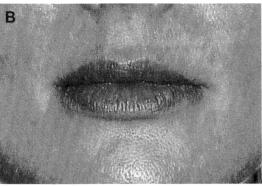

Fig. 20. Enhancement of lip volume with fat grafting. Fat grafting the lips produces a soft, natural-appearing improvement in lip appearance and slight undercorrection that is appropriate for the typical patient having a facelift and in need of enhanced lip volume. Nonautologous fillers invite overcorrection and tend to produce a more stylized lip appearance. (*A*) Perioral area of a patient having a facelift seen before fat grafting. (*B*) Same patient seen after facelift that included fat grafting of the lips. The lips are fuller and healthier appearing, but soft and natural looking. (*Courtesy of* Marten Clinic of Plastic Surgery. All surgical procedures performed by Timothy J. Marten, MD, FACS, San Francisco, CA.)

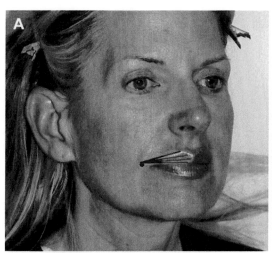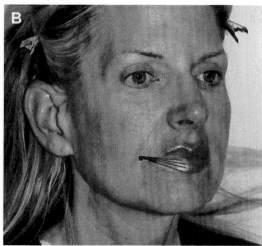

Fig. 21. Incision sites and plan for injecting fat into the upper and lower lip areas. Fat grafting of the lips is performed with a 5-cm, 0.7-mm (22-gauge) cannula and fat is placed submucosally beneath the vermillion and subdermally in the white-roll areas. Typically a total of 1 to 1.5 mL is placed in each side of the upper lip (*A*) and 1.5 to 2 mL are placed in each side of the lower lip (*B*).

perioral pucker lines in that these procedures only address the skin, and do nothing to replenish age-associated loss of perioral subcutaneous fat. Fat grafting provides a means by which outcomes can be improved and fat normally situated between skin and orbicularis oris muscle near the vermillion-cutaneous junction can be replenished. Experience with combined dermabrasion or laser resurfacing and perioral fat injections suggests that healing and the overall outcome are better when resurfacing procedures are combined with fat grafting, beyond the improvement gained by simple volume addition, and this may be attributable to a "stem cell effect" (**Fig. 22**).

When injecting the perioral area, care must be taken not to mistakenly overfill the white upper lip (area between the base of the nose and the vermillion-cutaneous junction) in a well-intended but misguided attempt to reduce upper lip wrinkles because patients' upper lips can be lengthened, dental show can be reduced, and abnormal convex simian contours in profile can result. A better strategy is to concentrate efforts on and near the white-roll area, where the wrinkles are typically the deepest and appear most objectionable, and place the most fat in this area. Less fat is then placed more superiorly. Injection in the perioral area is made with a 5 cm long, 0.7-mm (22-gauge) injection cannula in a subcutaneous/premuscular plane. Placing the fat deeper and intramuscularly is not helpful in creating the type of improvement that is usually sought in this area. Fat grafting the perioral area is intermediate to advanced in difficulty.

Jawline Fat grafting of the jawline can enhance patients' facial shapes and produce the kind of improvements obtained when mandibular border and Taylor-style mandibular angle implants are placed (**Fig. 23**).

Fat grafting along the mandible can also correct an atrophic and feeble appearance that occurs as the mandibular border shrinks with age by broadening and strengthening it. Treatment of the jawline typically must be undertaken in conjunction with the GMG and the two areas overlap in most cases.

Fat grafting of the jawline is typically performed with an 8 cm long, 1.2-mm (18-gauge) injection cannula from injection sites on the perioral area and mandibular border (**Fig. 24**) and fat is placed deep in a preperiosteal/submasseteric position on the surface of the bone.

Between 3 and 6 mL of fat are typically placed on each side depending on the deficiency present, but occasionally more is indicated. Note that fat is not injected subcutaneously, into the parotid, or into the masseter muscle.

Although not intuitively obvious, strengthening the jawline and posterior mandibular border makes the patient appear more youthful, fit, and attractive, and is an artistically powerful adjunct to a facelift that helps avert the deficient, frail, and lackluster mandibular contour typically seen in aging and elderly faces that is usually made worse when a facelift is performed (discussed later).

Fat grafting the jawline is particularly useful in patients having secondary facelifts and in patients

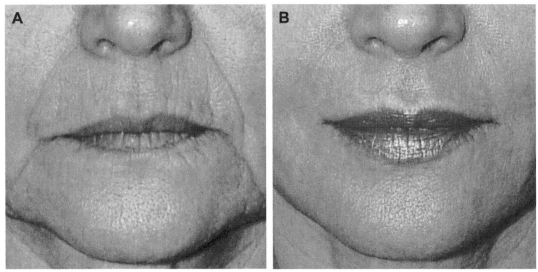

Fig. 22. Combined perioral dermabrasion and fat grafting. (*A*) Patient seen preoperatively with wrinkled, atrophic perioral area that lends an elderly, unhealthy, and objectionable appearance to the face. (*B*) Same patient seen 2 years and 7 months after high SMAS facelift that included combined perioral fat grafting and perioral dermabrasion. Both atrophy and wrinkling have been improved, and the mouth has a more youthful, healthy, and kissable appearance. The combined treatment produced a better appearance than either procedure performed alone. (*Courtesy of* Marten Clinic of Plastic Surgery. All surgical procedures performed by Timothy J. Marten, MD, FACS, San Francisco, CA.)

with long faces seeking facial rejuvenation or improvement. Fat grafting of this area allows the face to be broadened, and overall proportions improved (**Fig. 25**). Fat grafting the jawline area is intermediate in difficulty.

Temple area Temporal hollowing is consistently seen by the fourth decade of life and beyond in most patients seeking facial rejuvenation and can be readily improved with fat grafting (**Fig. 26**).

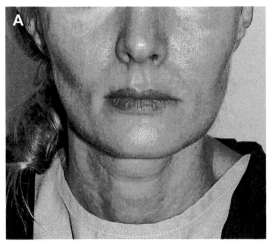
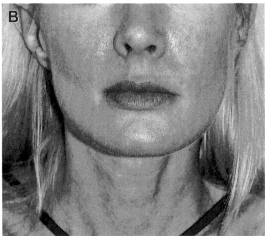

Fig. 23. Using fat grafting to enhance mandibular contour and strengthen the jawline. (*A*) Patient seen before surgery with small mandible, narrow intergonial distance, and lower facial disproportion. (*B*) Same patient after high SMAS facelift and fat grafting of the posterior jawline. No implants have been placed. Strengthening the jawline and posterior mandibular border results in a more fit and proportionate appearance, and helps avert the tight and deficient mandibular contour typically seen in the elderly face after a facelift is performed (note: fat has also been injected in the chin, GMGs, buccal recess, and lip areas). (*Courtesy of* Marten Clinic of Plastic Surgery. All surgical procedures performed by Timothy J. Marten, MD, FACS, San Francisco, CA.)

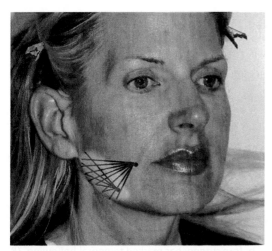

Fig. 24. Incision sites and plan for injecting fat into the posterior jawline. Fat grafting of the jawline is usually performed with an 8-cm, 1.2-mm (18-gauge) cannula and fat is placed in a preperiosteal/submasseteric position. Typically 3 to 6 mL of fat are placed in each side. Note that fat is not injected subcutaneously, into the parotid, or into the masseter muscle. Level of difficulty: intermediate.

The temple areas are grafted in a subcutaneous plane from small stab incisions just within the temporal hairline (**Fig. 27**) if a forehead lift is simultaneously being performed that requires dissection in the temporal subgaleal plane. If a temporal subgaleal dissection is not performed as part of the procedure, injection can be made superficially and deep.

Between 5 and 7 mL of fat are typically placed in the temple area on each side, but occasionally more is indicated. In most cases a slightly larger diameter and blunter 0.9-mm (20-gauge), 6 cm long injection cannula is superior to sharper and smaller types that are preferred elsewhere. Using a slightly larger diameter cannula helps avoid perforation of temporal veins that are predictably present in the temporal area and allows fat to be placed over and around them to conceal them.

When treating the temple area, the injection cannula is not passed specifically above or below the temporal veins when present but is allowed to pass into the plane of least resistance in the subcutaneous plane. Experience has shown this to be an excellent strategy, and one that is less likely to injure temporal veins. Should a temporal vein accidentally be perforated during temple injection despite these precautions and swelling from the leakage of venous blood noted, it is a simple matter to hold pressure on the temporal area for a few moments with a surgical sponge. Typically after applying uniform and continuous pressure for a few minutes, bleeding stops and treatment of the area can be completed. Fat grafting the temple areas is intermediate in difficulty.

Buccal recess area Buccal atrophy is consistently seen in the fourth decade of life and beyond, as is buccal hollowing caused by previous overzealous excision of buccal fat, or human immunodeficiency virus–associated facial wasting (**Fig. 28**).

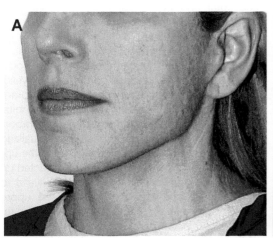

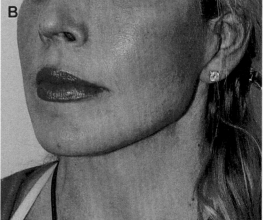

Fig. 25. Using fat grafting to broaden the face and correct the long face disproportion. (*A*) Preoperative view of patient with a small mandible and long face. A previous facelift performed by an unknown surgeon has tightened the mandibular line and accentuated facial length. (*B*) Same patient seen after fat grafting of the jawline, chin, cheeks, midface, buccal recess, and lip areas. No implants have been placed. The long appearance has been improved and a more balanced and proportionate look has been obtained. (*Courtesy of* Marten Clinic of Plastic Surgery. All surgical procedures performed by Timothy J. Marten, MD, FACS, San Francisco, CA.)

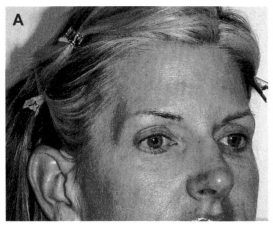
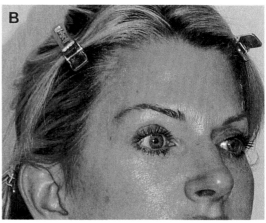

Fig. 26. Filling of the temple hollow with fat. Temporal hollowing is a consistent marker of the fourth decade of life that can readily be improved by fat grafting. (*A*) Patient before surgery has marked temporal hollowing. (*B*) Same patient after high SMAS facelift and fat grafting of the temple region (note: fat has also been injected in the upper and lower orbital areas). (*Courtesy of* Marten Clinic of Plastic Surgery. All surgical procedures performed by Timothy J. Marten, MD, FACS, San Francisco, CA.)

Fat grafting of the buccal hollow is typically performed with a 4 cm long, 0.7-mm (22-gauge) injection cannula from injection sites situated on the midface and medial lower cheek (**Fig. 29**) and fat is placed subcutaneously and in sub-SMAS (buccal space) locations.

Between 2 and 5 mL of fat are typically placed on each side in the buccal recess area, depending on the degree of the problem, but occasionally more is indicated. Often an asymmetrical placement of fat is also required on the right and left sides because of the common occurrence of

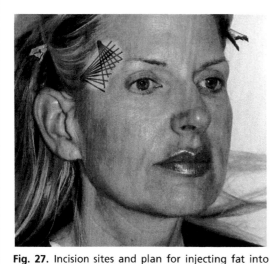

Fig. 27. Incision sites and plan for injecting fat into the temple areas. Fat grafting of the temples is performed with a 5-cm, 0.9-mm (20-gauge) cannula and fat is placed in a subcutaneous and/or deep plane depending on whether a temporal subgaleal dissection is made. Typically 5 to 7 mL of fat are placed on each side. Level of difficulty: intermediate.

buccal asymmetry seen preoperatively in many patients. Fat grafting the buccal recess area is intermediate in difficulty.

Upper orbit/upper eyelid area Whether the result of illness, aging, or previous overzealous surgical treatment, filling the hollow upper orbit can produce a rejuvenation of the upper eyelid and eliminate an unnaturally hollow and elderly appearance, sometimes referred to by patients as nursing-home or owl eyes (**Fig. 30**).

Where fat should be placed in the upper orbit (upper eyelid) is a subject of debate, but for all but very experienced injectors it is safest to avoid subseptal and purely subcutaneous injections, and limit initial grafting to a preperiosteal/sub–orbicularis oculi plane.

A common misconception in treating hollow upper orbits is that the fat is needed and should be grafted into the preseptal portion of the eyelid. Hollow upper eyelids are more properly and practically restored by placing fat in a preorbital position along the inferior margins of the supraorbital rim and the process is best conceptualized as lowering the supraorbital rim and filling the upper orbital area to push skin that has retracted up into the orbit down onto the preseptal eyelid to create a full and appropriately creased upper eyelid. Once the surgeon accepts that improvement is obtained by grafting of the orbit, and not of the eyelid, it becomes apparent that larger volumes than might otherwise be expected are required. In general, 2 to 3 mL of fat must be placed on each side in each upper orbit to achieve the improvement that is typically sought. Smaller injection cannulas are now available and have

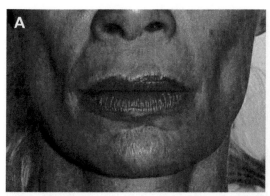
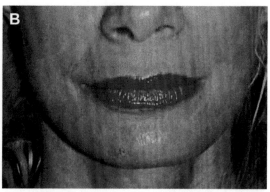

Fig. 28. Correction of buccal atrophy and overexcision of buccal fat. Buccal fat excision is often erroneously recommended as a way of creating a high cheekbone and more angular facial appearance. In reality, it often produces an ill, haggard, gaunt, and unfeminine appearance, especially when performed aggressively. (*A*) Patient with buccal hollowing following buccal fat excision by an unknown surgeon. (*B*) Same patient after fat grafting of the buccal area (note: fat has also been placed in the infraorbital, midface, cheek, preoral, and jawline areas). (*Courtesy of* Marten Clinic of Plastic Surgery. All surgical procedures performed by Timothy J. Marten, MD, FACS, San Francisco, CA.)

made injecting the upper orbit easier and more predictable than in the past because they can be advanced more smoothly and accurately through tissues and allow the deposition of very tiny aliquots of fat on each pass. At present, a 4 cm long, 0.7-mm (22-gauge) cannula is preferred.

When grafting the upper orbit it must always be remembered that the surgeon is working in close proximity to the eye and, although the injection cannulas are blunt tipped, they are easily capable of perforating the ocular globe.

Fat grafting the upper orbit and eyelid is advanced in difficulty and treatment of this area

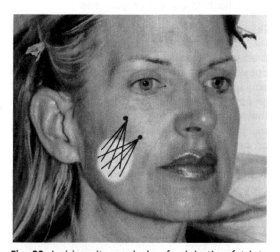

Fig. 29. Incision sites and plan for injecting fat into the buccal hollows. Fat grafting of the buccal hollow is typically performed with a 4–cm, 0.7-mm (22-gauge) cannula and fat is placed subcutaneously and in sub-SMAS (buccal space) locations in most cases. Typically 2 to 5 mL of fat are placed in each side. Level of difficulty: intermediate.

should be attempted only after experience has been gained in treating more forgiving areas (**Fig. 31**). Once that experience is obtained, fat grafting the upper orbit can be one of the most artistically rewarding uses of autologous fat, and one that is likely to become a routine part of rejuvenating the upper eyelid in the future.

Lower orbit/lower eyelid area Injecting the infraorbital (lower eyelid) area is in many ways analogous to injecting the upper orbit in that there are similar misconceptions as to where the fat should be placed, similar technical considerations as to where fat should be injected, and similar concerns regarding injury to the ocular globe. In addition, and like fat grafting the upper orbit, the artistic payoff is high if the procedure is performed carefully and correctly (**Fig. 32**).

Fat grafting the infraorbital area allows comprehensive correction of age-associated hollowness that lends the face an ill or haggard appearance, shortens the apparent length of the lower eyelid, and produces a youthful, attractive, and highly desirable smooth transition from the lower eyelid to the cheek that is generally unobtainable by traditional lower eyelid surgery, fat transpositions, septal resets, midface lifts, free fat grafts, and other like means. As is the case in treating the upper orbit, fat need not and should not be grafted in the pretarsal lower eyelid. Fat should be injected deep in a submuscular/preperiosteal plane, and the technical goal of the procedure should be thought of as raising up and anteriorly projecting the infraorbital rim rather than filling the lid itself. Like the upper orbit, volumes required to obtain corrections in the lower orbit are typically more than might initially be expected, and 2 to 3 mL

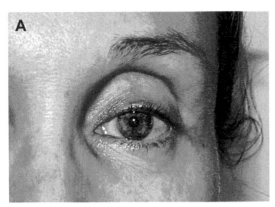
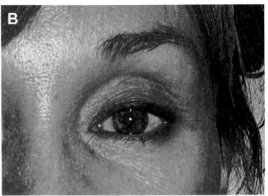

Fig. 30. Correcting upper orbital hollowing. (*A*) Patient with hollow upper eyelid and unnaturally hollow ocular appearance (owl eyes) following blepharoplasty performed by an unknown surgeon. (*B*) Same patient seen after fat grafting of the upper orbit. A healthier, more youthful appearance can be seen. (*Courtesy of* Marten Clinic of Plastic Surgery. All surgical procedures performed by Timothy J. Marten, MD, FACS, San Francisco, CA.)

per side are necessary to produce the desired effect in most cases, and occasionally more. However, unlike the upper orbit, experience has shown that fat is best and most easily injected perpendicular to the infraorbital rim, and, when this is done, lumps and irregularities are far less common. Fat should not be injected parallel to the lid-cheek junction in the infraorbital area.

Fat grafting of the infraorbital area is typically performed with a 4 cm long, 0.7-mm (22-gauge) injection cannula from injection sites in the mid-cheek or perioral area (**Fig. 33**).

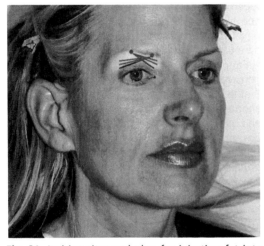

Fig. 31. Incision sites and plan for injecting fat into the upper orbital (upper eyelid) area. Fat grafting of the upper orbital area is typically performed with a 4-cm, 0.7-mm (22-gauge) cannula and fat is placed deep in a sub–orbicularis oculi/preperiosteal plane. Typically 2 to 3 mL of fat are placed on each side in each upper orbit. Level of difficulty: advanced.

As is the case in grafting the upper orbit, when grafting the lower orbit the surgeon should place the index fingers of the nondominant (noninjecting) hand firmly on the infraorbital rim to protect the ocular globe while injections are made.

It is wise to avoid any subcutaneous injection in the infraorbital area because of the extremely thin skin present and the likelihood of creating visible lumps and irregularities, and to limit grafting to a preperiosteal/sub–orbicularis oculi plane. The purported benefits of superficial grafting (improving skin texture and color) are too small an improvement in most cases for all but expert injectors to offset the likely occurrence of visible and difficult-to-correct irregularities.

Tear trough Where the infraorbital area ends and the tear trough and cheek areas begin is hard to precisely define; the treatment of the infraorbital, cheek, and tear trough areas must be undertaken concurrently in most patients, and the treated areas overlap each other to a certain extent, as they do on other areas of the face. In addition, it must always be remembered that the goal of the procedure is creating youthful and attractive contour, not simply filling a specific area.

Treatment of the tear tough is most easily and best performed using incisions situated inferior to the medial orbit and placing fat predominantly perpendicularly, as in the cheek and intraorbital areas (**Fig. 34**).

A 4 cm long, 0.7-mm (22-gauge) cannula is typically used and fat is placed deep in a preperiosteal/sub–orbicularis oculi plane, especially superiorly and medially, where the skin is the thinnest. As experience is gained, and if care is taken, fat can safely be placed more superficially, especially in the lower, more lateral part

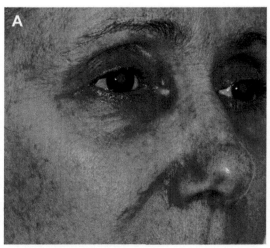
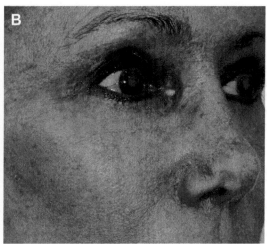

Fig. 32. Filling the hollow lower orbit with fat. (*A*) Patient with hollow lower eyelid and unnaturally hollow and elderly infraorbital appearance. The lower eyelid appears long and there is a distinct line of demarcation between the lower eyelid and the cheek. (*B*) Same patient seen after facelift and fat grafting of the infraorbital area. There is a smooth transition from the lower eyelid to the cheek and the patient has a more healthy, youthful, and attractive appearance (note: the upper orbit, radix, cheek, and nasolabial crease have also been treated with fat grafts and the patient has undergone ptosis correction). (*Courtesy of* Marten Clinic of Plastic Surgery. All surgical procedures performed by Timothy J. Marten, MD, FACS, San Francisco, CA.)

of the tear trough that is frequently seen to run down into and onto the cheek, and when this is done improved outcomes are obtained. From 0.5 to 1.5 mL of fat are typically placed on each side in the tear trough area, depending on how far inferiorly and laterally it extends onto the cheek (**Fig. 35**).

Although ostensibly seeming simple, fat grafting the tear trough is advanced in difficulty.

Final Touches

Fat grafting is continued until the indicated volume of fat has been added to each target area. Treated

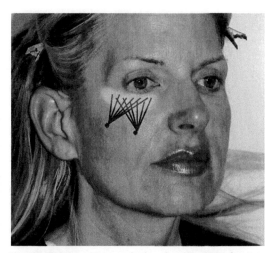
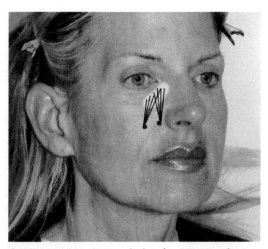

Fig. 33. Incision sites and plan for injecting fat into infraorbital (lower eyelid) area. Fat grafting of the infraorbital area is typically performed with a 4-cm, 0.7-mm (22-gauge) cannula and fat is placed deep in a sub–orbicularis oculi/preperiosteal plane. Typically 2 to 3 mL of fat are placed on each side, although occasionally more is needed. Level of difficulty: advanced.

Fig. 34. Incision sites and plan for injecting fat into the nasojugal (tear trough) areas. Fat grafting of the nasojugal tear trough area is typically performed with a 4-cm, 0.7-mm (22-gauge) injection cannula and fat is placed deep in a preperiosteal/sub–orbicularis oculi plane. Typically 0.5 to 1.5 mL of fat are placed on each side depending on how far inferiorly and laterally the tear trough extends onto the cheek. Level of difficulty: advanced.

areas are then gently palpated after they are injected to ensure that the fat has been distributed smoothly in the target tissue, and any lumps or irregularities are gently pressed out. The lips, stomal angle, and nasolabial areas can be bidigitally palpated and molded by inserting a gloved finger inside the mouth, and if the orbits have been treated the ocular globe should be gently depressed and irregularities checked for in the orbital area.

Documenting What was Done

A member of the operating room team should keep a detailed record of areas treated and amounts of fat injected in each area, and a fat injection treatment record is useful for this purpose (**Fig. 36**).

Typically a mark is entered on the record for each 1-mL syringe injected. In the absence of a circulating nurse, a copy of this record can be sterilized and a temporary tally of the fat injected kept by a scrubbed member of the operating room team using a sterile surgical marker (**Fig. 37**). The information recorded can later be transcribed to the patient's official (nonsterile) fat injection treatment record after the procedure has been completed.

Alternatively, amounts injected can be recorded by a nonscrubbed team member on life-sized laser print photographs of the patients face.

Learning the fat injection procedure

- Acknowledge atrophy as part of the aging deformity
- Learn the basics of the fat injection technique and obtain the needed equipment to properly perform the procedure
- Make the needed commitment of time to properly perform the procedure
- Do not underestimate the technical and artistic difficulty of the procedure
- Make small additions at first to gain familiarity with the technique
- Critically analyze outcomes
- Improve

Completion of Concurrently Planned Procedures

Once fat grafting is complete, attention is turned to the face, neck, and forehead, and upper blepharoplasty, lower blepharoplasty, perioral dermabrasion, and other planned procedures are performed as indicated. Because most fat is needed and will be grafted in the anterior face and other areas that do not overlap the areas dissected in these other procedures, performing them after fat is injected does not interfere significantly with their performance or compromise outcomes.

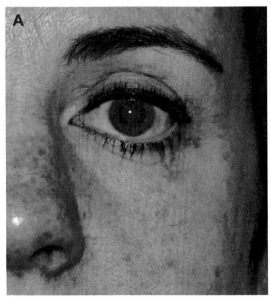
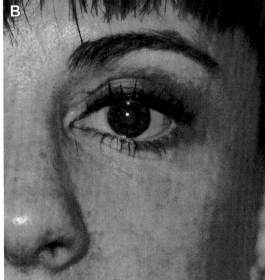

Fig. 35. Filling the tear trough with fat. (*A*) Patient with hollow nasojugal groove (tear trough) and unnaturally hollow and elderly infraorbital appearance. (*B*) Same patient seen after fat grafting. A more healthy and youthful ocular appearance is noted. (*Courtesy of* Marten Clinic of Plastic Surgery. All surgical procedures performed by Timothy J. Marten, MD, FACS, San Francisco, CA.)

Marten Clinic of Plastic Surgery
450 Sutter St Suite 2222 San Francisco, CA 94108

place patient sticker here

FAT INJECTION DATA SHEET

patient weight (lbs/kg) ______________

FAT INJECTION SITE:	**RIGHT**		**LEFT**
forehead	______		______
temples	______		______
glabella		______	
radix		______	
brow/ supra-orbital	______		______
infra-orbital	______		______
tear trough	______		______
mid-face	______		______
cheek	______		______
pre-auricular	______		______
buccal recess	______		______
nasolabial crease	______		______
piroform / nasal base	______		______
columella / nasolabial angle		______	
upper lip	______		______
lower lip	______		______
stomal angle	______		______
GMG / peri-mental	______		______
chin	______		______
jawline	______		______
labiomental (chin) crease		______	
submental crease		______	
misc intra-dermal		______	
other (list)			
	______		______
	______		______
	______		______
	______		______

Total Fat Injected - Face ______________

FAT HARVEST SITE (check all that apply)

- ❒ outer thighs
- ❒ hips
- ❒ inner thighs
- ❒ knees
- ❒ abdomen
- ❒ anterior thighs
- ❒ waist/flank
- ❒ other (list)

FAT HARVEST DATA

total fat harvested (cc) ______________

total fat after centrifuging (cc) ______________

centrifuge time ❒ 3 minutes
❒ ____ minutes

centrifuge speed
❒ _____ RPM

______________________ nurse signature

______________ date

Fig. 36. Fat injection data sheet. Using a fat injection data sheet simplifies the documentation of what was done and provides a clear and easily accessible record of the patient's treatment.

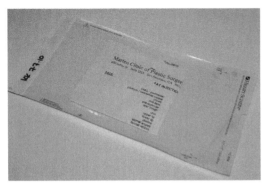

Fig. 37. Fat injection data sheet. The fat injection data sheet can be sterilized and a temporary record of the fat injected kept by a scrubbed member of the surgical team using a sterile surgical marker. The information can later be transcribed to the patient's medical record after the procedure has been completed.

Dressings

After all planned procedures have been completed and all incisions have been closed, the patient's hair is washed with shampoo, and rinsed. No dressing is required or applied.

POSTOPERATIVE CARE

Most patients having combined face lifts and fat grafting are discharged to an aftercare specialist the first night after surgery with specific written instructions as to how they are to care for the patient. Patients are asked to rest quietly and apply cool (but not ice or ice cold) compresses to their faces for 15 to 20 minutes of every hour they are awake for the first 3 days after surgery, or use a commercially available thermostatically regulated water-cooled mask (www.aqueductmedical. com). For most patients, edema peaks at about this time. Patients are advised not to place ice or ice-cold compresses on their faces because this is likely to damage grafted fat and to compromise outcomes.

Patients undergoing facelift and fat grafting are instructed to sleep flat on their backs without a pillow. A small cylindrical neck roll is permitted if the patient requests it. This position ensures an open cervicomental angle and averts the neck flexion that often results when a pillow is used. In addition, in this position swelling drains to the back of the head instead of the jowl, neck, and submental region where it is less harmful, less noticeable, and more rapidly transmitted away from the face to the torso when the patient sits upright.

Patients are advised to take a soft diet that is easy to chew and digest for 2 weeks after surgery, and are encouraged to avoid salty, dry foods that are difficult to chew.

RECOVERY AND HEALING

When patients return to work and their social lives depends on how aggressively their procedure was performed (how much fat was injected), their tolerance for surgery, their capacity for healing, the type of work they do, the activities they enjoy, their need for secrecy, and their overall opinion about their appearance. Patients are asked to set aside 2 to 3 weeks to recover from surgery, and additional time off is recommended before an important business presentation, family gathering, vacation, or similar event.

It is important for patient to know that fat grafting significantly increases facial swelling and often adds several weeks to their overall recovery. In some cases swelling even persists longer and is troubling for a longer period of time. Swelling is most pronounced and noticeable in the lips and eye areas. Patients having their lips fat grafted are given a cone-type surgical face mask and are encouraged to use it to conceal swelling in the mouth area in the early postoperative period. Ecchymosis is generally light and less of an issue for most patients than swelling and edema.

Patients are informed that it often takes 2 to 3 months to have a natural appearance in a photograph or to be seen at an important function. They are also advised to expect some firmness in the face and submental areas for 6 to 9 months.

Patients often mistakenly interpret the resolution of swelling and the return of some facial wrinkles as poor fat graft survival, and often comment once healing is complete that "the fat went away". Such comments arise out of the joy most patients experience when they see their faces full and smooth initially after the procedure, because volume addition to the face often produces subtle three-dimensional changes, and because most patients simply forget the extent to which a lack of volume was present in the treated areas on their preoperative faces. Treating surgeons can also sometimes initially experience similar disappointment for similar reasons, and it can take time to learn to recognize the improvements that are made.

RETREATMENT

Most of the change in facial contour seen on patients' faces 4 to 6 months after their procedures is likely to consist of living fat and represent a persistent improvement, and patients can be informed that most of what they see is what they get at that point because swelling and induration have mostly abated by that time. Four to 6 months after surgery is also the time at which most surgeons performing fat grafting think that facial edema, induration, and inflammation have resolved sufficiently for retreatment to be considered if it is indicated and the patient requests it. Because there is a limit to the amount of fat that can be infiltrated properly into a thin atrophic face, the need for secondary, second-stage fat grafting should not be viewed as a failure of the primary procedure; it is simply an inherent limitation of the technique. If the patient achieved improvement with the primary treatment, a secondary procedure will typically be equally or more beneficial, and often need to be far less comprehensive than the first.

COMPLICATIONS

No major complications attributable to fat grafting, including infection, embolization, tissue infarction, or blindness, have been seen while performing the procedure simultaneously with facelifts over the last 20 years. However, these problems have been reported and are known to occur when fat grafting is performed. Clinical experience has shown that embolization is extremely uncommon when fat infiltration is made with a blunt cannula, but this could change as infiltration cannulas become smaller and more surgeons perform the procedure. Embolization and related complications, including blindness, are largely attributable to sharp needle injection, and these and other complications of fat grafting have been discussed in detail by Coleman[13] and others.

Complications of simultaneous facelift and fat grafting attributable to the fat injection procedure are largely minor and aesthetic problems and include lumps, oil cysts, asymmetries, undercorrection, overcorrection, and donor site irregularities. However, these are more accurately considered inherent risks of the procedure, much like breast implant encapsulization, in that even if the procedure is technically performed properly and with care the variations in take that can occur with any graft and that are beyond the surgeon's control can cause them. This consideration is particularly true in the case of fat grafts, because fat tissue is fragile.

Certain patients seem to be at higher risk for problems and complications, largely owing to the compromised condition of fat donor and recipient sites. Such patients include smokers and former smokers; patients who have undergone previous facial liposuction; patients who have had radiation therapy; and patients who have undergone intense pulsed light, radiofrequency, and ultrasonography skin-shrinking treatments. Unlike laser resurfacing procedures in which energy is dispersed on the skin surface, these pulsed light, radiofrequency,

and ultrasonic procedures disperse energy in the deep dermis and subcutaneous areas and can cause damage to tissue microcirculation that seems to compromise graft take. Compromise of a similar sort also seems to be present in patients who have had large volumes of inflammatory fillers (poly-L-lactic acid [PLLA], calcium phosphate, and so forth) and in patients who have had large volumes of hyaluronic acid (HA)–based fillers present for a long time. Simply dissolving HA fillers enzymatically with hyaluronidase does not seem to eliminate this problem because residual inflammation seems to still be present and can result in suboptimal graft take. All such patients should be approached with caution, and they should know that they are likely to be at an increased risk of problems and complications.

Patients who have undergone previous liposuction, especially laser or ultrasonic types, are typically more difficult to harvest fat from, and the fat harvested typically has an increased oil (ruptured fat cell) fraction and is more likely to have fibrotic tissue fragments that clog injection cannulas.

Most complications are small and easily managed if fat grafting is performed properly and conservative additions of fat are made. Oil cysts can usually simply be aspirated or unroofed. Lumps have been exceedingly rare in our own experience, but are now being increasingly seen in patients treated by other physicians. These lumps can usually be treated by microliposuction, direct excision, or overgrafting with more fat. Asymmetries and undercorrections are generally treatable by additional fat grafting, and donor site irregularities with touch-up liposuction and/or fat grafts. Overcorrection is uncommon in single-stage treatments and is typically seen in patients who have undergone multiple fat grafting procedures. Other than in the orbital and lip areas, when overcorrection occurs improvement can be made by judicious extraction of fat from overcorrected areas by a microliposuction technique using a 0.9-mm or 0.7-mm cannula attached to a 3-mL syringe. Irregularities or overfilling of the orbital areas are best treated by opening the eyelid and removing offending fat under direct vision, and small lumps and bumps on the lips are readily treated by direct excision using a radially situated incision made in a vermillion wrinkle.

The best way to treat complications is to avoid them, and the surgeons experiencing the fewest problems are likely to be the ones who take the time to learn to perform the procedure properly, obtain the needed equipment necessary to do so, and who introduce it into their practice gradually and in a conservative manner.

SUMMARY

Recognizing the changes that occur as the face ages and appreciating the underlying anatomic problems responsible for them is essential to properly advising patients and to planning surgical procedures. In most patients, problems are in 3 general categories: (1) aging and breakdown of the skin surface; (2) tissue sagging, skin redundancy, and loss of youthful facial contour; and (3) facial hollowing and atrophy. Skin care and skin resurfacing procedures address changes in the first category. The traditional lifts of the face, neck, forehead, and eyes address the second. Fat grafting allows clinicians to treat atrophy, something they have previously been unable to do, and fat grafting is now acknowledged by surgeons treating the aging face as the most important advance in aesthetic surgery in several decades or more. Properly performed, the addition of fat to areas of the face that have atrophied because of age can produce a significant and sustained improvement in appearance that is unobtainable by other means.

CASE EXAMPLES

Patient Example 1

Shown are before-after surgery views of woman, aged 45 years. The patient has had no previous plastic surgery.

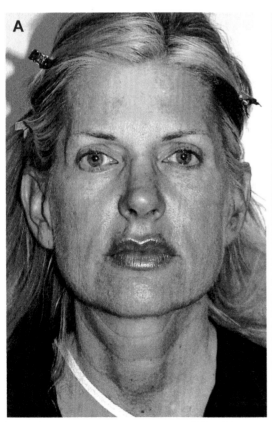 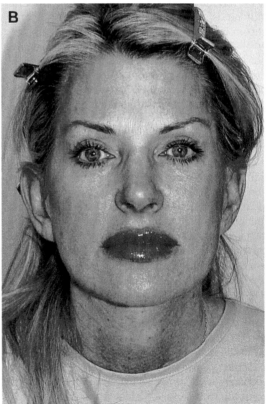

(*A, C, E*) Pre-surgery views 1. Note overall facial laxity and panfacial atrophy. (*B, D, F*) Same patient, 2 years and 4 months after high SMAS facelift, neck lift, closed forehead lift, lower eyelift, and fat transfer to the temples, cheeks, lips, nasolabial, GMG, stomal angles, and upper and lower eye lid areas (see Fig. 2 for fat placement). A total of 50 mL of fat was placed. Note soft, natural facial contours and the absence of a tight, pulled, or face-lifted appearance. Facial atrophy has also been simultaneously corrected and the patient has a healthier, more youthful, and more feminine appearance. The combined facelift and fat injection procedures have produced a result that arguably could not be obtained by either procedure alone. (*Courtesy of* Marten Clinic of Plastic Surgery).

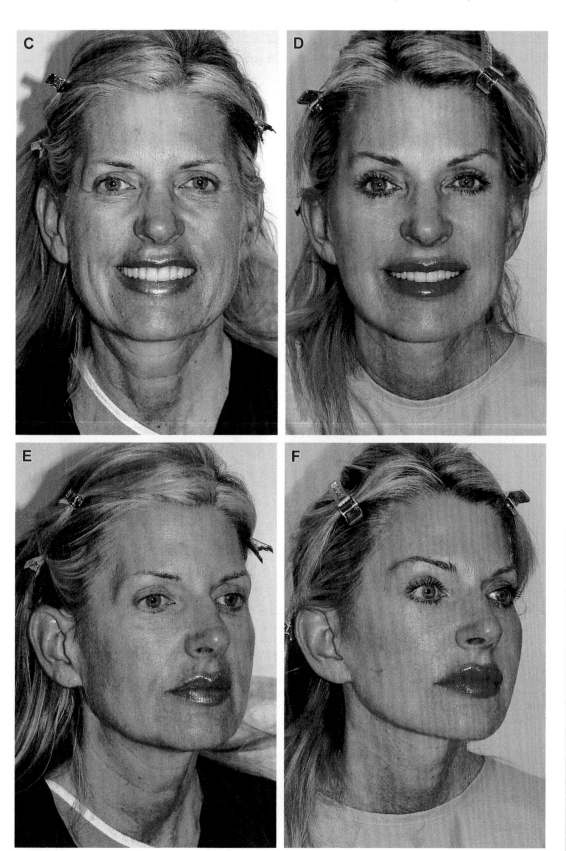

Patient Example 2

Shown are before-after surgery views of man, aged 68 years.

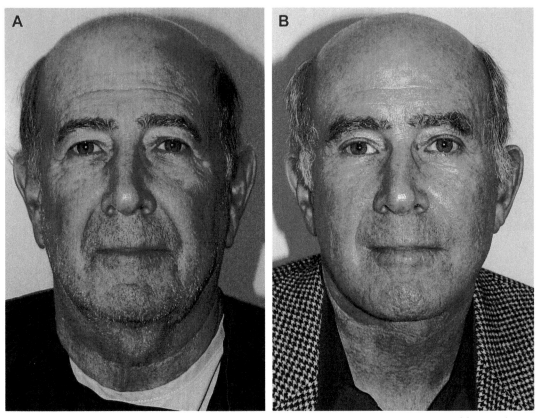

(*A, C, E*) Pre-surgery views 1. The patient has sagging cheeks, deep cheek folds, and jowls. Loss of facial volume is also evident in the cheeks, infraorbital, and perioral and GMG areas. (*B, D, F*) Same patient, 1 year and 9 months after high SMAS facelift, neck lift, closed forehead lift, upper and lower eye lifts, partial facial fat grafting, and ear lobe reduction. A total of 28 mL of fat was placed. Note restoration of youthful and masculine facial shape without a tight or pulled appearance. Facial atrophy has also been simultaneously corrected and the patient has a healthier, more youthful, and more masculine appearance. The combined facelift and fat injection procedures have produced a result that arguably could not be obtained by either procedure alone. (*Courtesy of* Marten Clinic of Plastic Surgery. All surgical procedures performed by Timothy J. Marten, MD, FACS, San Francisco, CA.)

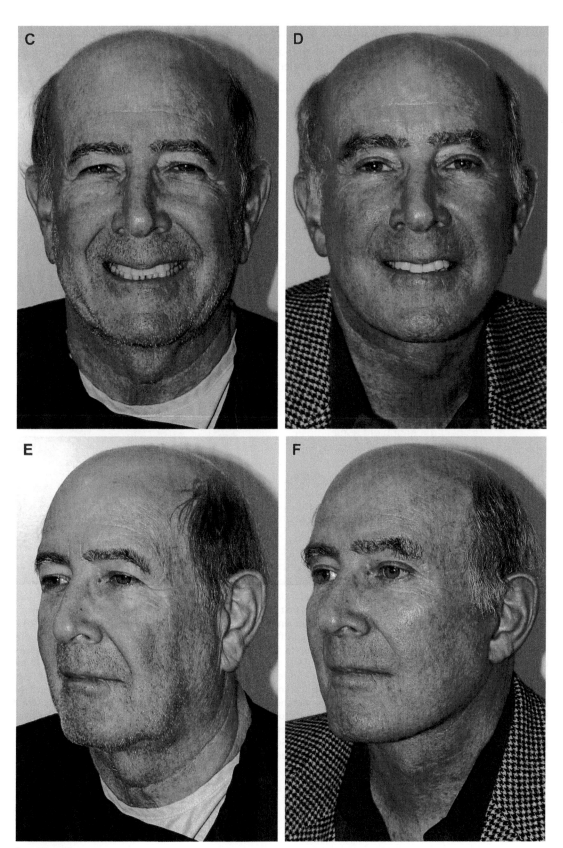

Patient Example 3

Shown are before-after surgery views of woman, aged 62 years. The patient has had previous facelift, neck lift, blepharoplasties, and other procedures performed by an unknown surgeon.

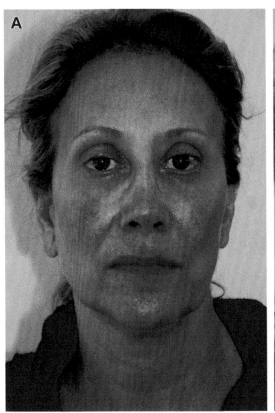
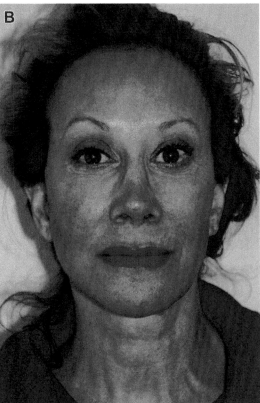

(*A, C, E*) Pre-surgery views 1. The patient has residual facial sagging and neck and jowl fullness following previous surgeries. Although the patient's face appears full at first glance, a careful examination shows regional atrophy in the temples, cheeks, and orbital, perioral, GMG, chin, and jawline areas. (*B, D, F*) Same patient, 12 months after high SMAS facelift, neck lift, small incision forehead lift, trichloroacetic acid (TCA) lower eyelid peel, ear lobe reduction, perioral dermabrasion, and fat transfer to the temples, glabella, radix, and upper orbital, lower orbital, cheek, midface, nasolabial, perioral, lips, GMG, stomal angle, chin, and jawline areas. A total of 70 mL of fat was placed simultaneously with the facelift and related procedures. Note the soft, natural facial contours and the absence of a tight, pulled, or facelifted appearance. Facial shape has been significantly improved and the patient now has a more youthful and healthy appearance. Although fat has been added to the patient's face it has a more trim, fit, and feminine appearance. Note also that the lips are fuller but natural appearing. The combined facelift and fat injection procedures have produced a result than arguably could not be obtained by either procedure alone. (*Courtesy of* Marten Clinic of Plastic Surgery. All surgical procedures performed by Timothy J. Marten, MD, FACS, San Francisco, CA. Previous procedures performed by an unknown surgeon.)

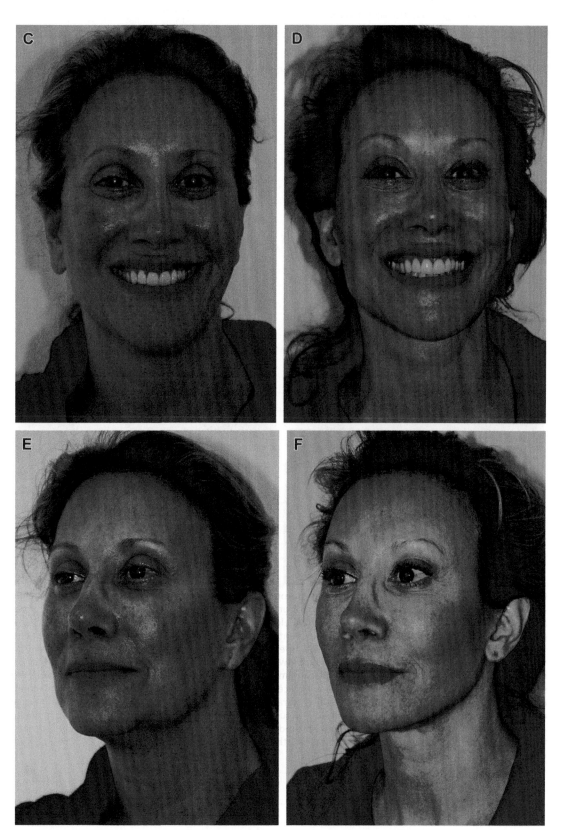

(continued)

Patient Example 4

Shown are before-after surgery views of a woman, aged 75 years. The patient has had multiple prior facelifts and related procedures, including previous laser resurfacing performed by unknown plastic surgeons.

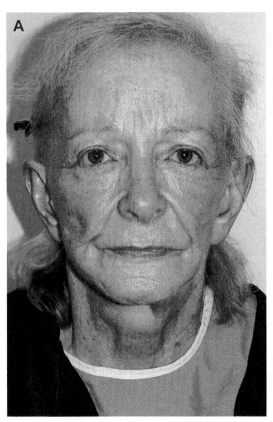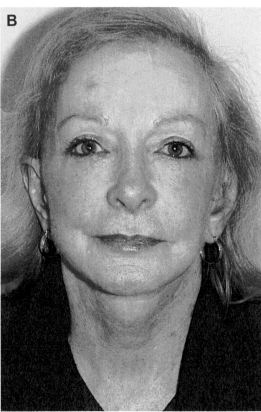

(*A, C, E*) Pre-surgery views 1. Preoperative views of a woman, aged 75 years, who has had multiple prior facelifts and related procedures, including previous laser resurfacing performed by unknown plastic surgeons. Note marked cheek laxity despite prior surgeries and frail, elderly appearance caused by uncorrected panfacial atrophy. Another facelift would predictably produce a gaunt, haggard, or even ill appearance. (*B, D, F*) Same patient, 1 year 7 months after high SMAS facelift, neck lift, forehead lift, upper and lower eyelifts, canthopexy, and fat transfer to the temples, cheeks, midface, upper and lower eyelids, lips, nasolabial creases, stomal angles, GMGs, chin, and jaw line. A total of 90 mL of fat was placed simultaneously with the facelift and related procedures. No skin resurfacing, facial implants, or other ancillary procedures were performed. In these situations fat injections and grafting are arguably more important to the overall outcome of the facelift than the facelift itself. Facial contour has been significantly enhanced, and facial volume restored. The patient has a healthy, fit, and feminine appearance that could not be obtained by either procedure performed alone. (*Courtesy of* Marten Clinic of Plastic Surgery. All surgical procedures performed by Timothy J. Marten, MD, FACS, San Francisco, CA. Previous procedures performed by an unknown surgeon.)

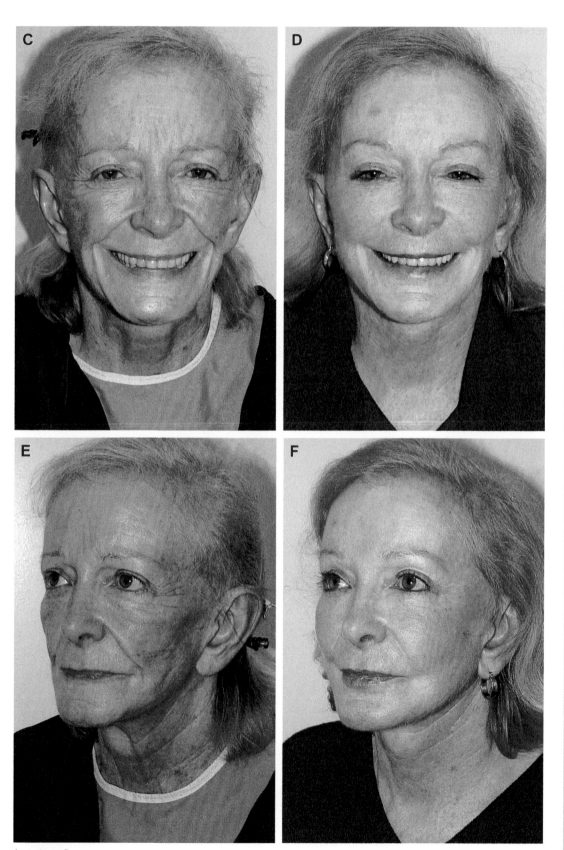

REFERENCES

1. Marten TJ. Simultaneous facelift and fat grafting: combined lifting and filling of the face. In: Nahai F, editor. Aesthetic plastic surgery. 2nd edition. 2011.
2. Marten TJ. Secondary facelift. In: Nelgin, editor. Plastic surgery. 2012.
3. Marten TJ. Lamellar high SMAS face and mid-lift: improved design of the SMAS facelift for better results in the mid-face and infra-orbital region. In: Nahai F, editor. Aesthetic plastic surgery. 2nd edition. 2011.
4. Marten TJ. Facelift. In: Guyuron B, editor. Plastic surgery: indications and practice. 2008.
5. Marten TJ. High SMAS facelift – combined single flap lifting of the jawline. Cheek, and midface. In: Paul M, editor. Clinics in plastic surgery. Elsevier; 2008.
6. Marten TJ. Secondary rejuvenation of the face. In: Mathes S, editor. Plastic surgery. Saunders-Elsevier; 2006.
7. Marten TJ. Maintenance facelift: early facelift for younger patients. In: Marten T, editor. Facelift: state of the art. Seminars in plastic surgery. New York: Thieme Medical Publishing; 2002.
8. Marten TJ. Facelift: planning and technique. In: Paul M, editors. Clinics in plastic surgery. 1997.
9. Connell BF, Marten TJ. Deep layer techniques in cervico-facial rejuvenation deep face-lifting. New York: Thieme Medical Publishers; 1994.
10. Connell BF, Marten TJ. Mastery of plastic and reconstructive surgery. New York: Little Brown Publishing; 1994.
11. Connell BF, Marten TJ. Surgical correction of the crow's feet deformity. Clin Plast Surg 1993;20(2): 295–302.
12. Connell BF, Marten TJ. Facelift for the active man. Instructional courses in plastic surgery. St Louis (MO): C.V. Mosby Co; 1991.
13. Coleman S. Structural fat grafting. 1st edition. 2004.

Gluteal Augmentation with Fat Grafting

The Brazilian Buttock Technique: 30 Years' Experience

 CrossMark

Luiz S. Toledo, MD

KEYWORDS

- Liposuction • Liposculpture • Fat grafting • Buttocks • Adipose tissue • Brazilian • Beauty

KEY POINTS

- This procedure is for increasing the projection of the gluteal region through the association of liposuction and fat grafting.
- There are 2 main body types: gynoid, with a concentration of fat below the waistline, and android, which concentrates fat above of the waistline.
- Both types can benefit from this type of surgery.
- The gynoid type in general needs liposuction of the hips, thighs, legs, and tummy and fat injection in the buttocks.
- The android type needs liposuction of the arms, axilla, back, hips, tummy, and breasts with fat injection of the buttocks and often the inner thighs as well.

HISTORY AND EVOLUTION OF FAT GRAFTING FOR BUTTOCK AUGMENTATION

Illouz[1] introduced liposuction in Brazil in November 1980, and Fournier[2] showed us liposculpture in 1983. We have been performing liposuction since 1982 and we learned from them that fat could be reinjected. In 1985, I started injecting large quantities of fat obtained from liposuction into different areas of the face and body. At the time other surgeons were injecting small quantities of fat on the face, 5 to 10 mL, into the malar areas and nasolabial folds or in the body to correct small liposuction sequelae. My work was the first to show the safety of injecting large quantities of fat in one surgical procedure. The area where the most quantity of fat was injected was the buttocks, up to 450 mL on each side.

At the time not many surgeons were using the liposculpture technique, and we had to find our way slowly. Soon we started injecting larger amounts in different areas of the body, 500 mL into each buttock, 300 mL in each breast, 300 mL into each medial thigh, and so forth. Patients were happy with the results, and we realized that with careful planning we could totally reshape the face and body by aspirating and injecting fat. We showed our results and published an abstract of our 18-month experience in 218 patients at the International Society of Aesthetic Plastic Surgery (ISAPS) Congress in New York City in 1987. We experienced for the first time from our peers the rejection that the fat grafting technique would suffer in the years to come. Criticism was usually concentrated on 2 points: the safety of patients and the reabsorption of the injected fat. The article "Eighteen Month Experience with Injected Fat Grafting" was published in 1988.[3]

In 1988, the only accepted procedure for volume augmentation was the insertion of silicone implants.

Disclosure: nothing to disclose.
Medical Arts Clinic, Dubai London Clinic, Saudi-German Hospital, PO Box 213522, Jumeirah, Dubai, United Arab Emirates
E-mail address: ToledoDubai@gmail.com

Clin Plastic Surg 42 (2015) 253–261
http://dx.doi.org/10.1016/j.cps.2014.12.004

Fat grafting had been discredited as a viable option since the time of Peer.[4] Peer had shown that fat grafts could have a survival rate of 50%. To some it was a failure. To others, like me, a 50% of survival of the graft was a success. I showed fat grafting could have major advantages with fewer complications.

By 1988 I had changed from the aspirator to syringes. I created the Brazilian Buttock technique, which consists of aspiration of fat from the flanks, abdomen, and thighs with injection into the buttocks and trochanter areas. Injected fat grafting undoubtedly constitutes a major step in repositioning the loss of soft tissue, which before was very difficult to correct.

In 1995, I performed surgical demonstrations of buttock augmentation at the University of Southern California (USC). The results were shown after 6 months in the United States at the Teleplast video-conference.[5] In 1996, I reported 8-year results with syringe liposculpture, for the treatment of localized fat deposits, to reshape the body and the face using disposable syringes and fine tip cannulas. In some cases, I inject up to 500 mL of fat on each side of the buttocks, in the muscle, on the muscle, into the fatty tissue, and subcutaneously, when needed. In the inner thigh, I have injected from 100 to 300 mL and in the calf from 50 to 150 mL. Fat grafting was performed in multiple tunnels in the deep and superficial planes. Fat absorption was estimated by clinical evaluation and measurements to be between 20% and 50% of the volume.[6]

Since then I have treated thousands of patients, performing facial and body augmentation. On the face, fat is injected to treat wrinkles and depressions, improve malars and zygomas, nasolabial and nasojugal folds, lips, and eyelids. In the body I perform buttock augmentation and reshaping, filling trochanteric depressions, breast augmentation, medial thighs augmentation, calf and ankle augmentation, treating liposuction sequelae, improving scar depressions, and hands and fingers. The technique of injection of liposuctioned fat, initially received with discredit, was accepted only after years of showing good results. Today it has become one of the hottest topics in most plastic surgery meetings.

AESTHETIC CONSIDERATIONS OF BUTTOCK AUGMENTATION

Normal buttocks should have a smooth round gluteal projection; a short intergluteal fold the infragluteal fold should reach the midthigh line. The waist-hip ratio (WHR) is a significant measure of female attractiveness (**Fig. 1**). Preferences may vary

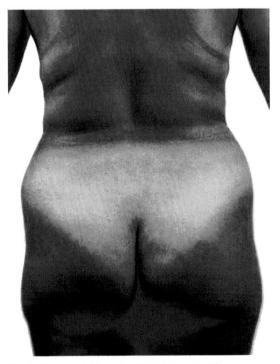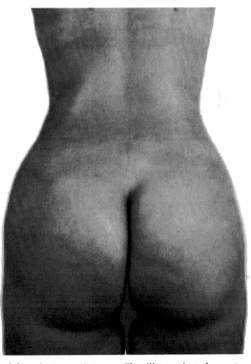

Fig. 1. The waist-hip ratio (WHR) is a significant measure of female attractiveness. The illustration shows two different patients. On the left a patient of the android type of body, with fat concentrated in the upper body. On the right a gynoid type patient, with fine waist and fat concentrated on the lower body. The lateral thighs should be in continuation with the shape of the buttock without excess fat. The back and flanks should not have excess fat and should have a smooth curve towards the buttocks.

according the ethnicity, but it is usually 0.6 in South America and 0.7 in European cultures. The lateral thighs should be in continuation with the shape of the buttock without excess fat. The back and flanks should not have excess fat and should have a smooth curve toward the buttocks. Usually buttock distortions happen because of flaccidity and ptosis, with accumulation of fat in the lower third of the buttock and forming a depression in the upper two-thirds. Usually 3 incisions are sufficient to treat the buttocks: one in the trochanter, one in the inter-gluteal fold, and one in the subgluteal fold. From these 3, I can aspirate and inject fat in all the areas (**Fig. 2**). I combine superficial liposuction in the lower third (when necessary) with fat grafting on the depressed areas, buttocks, and/or trochanter. Superficial irregularities can also happen because of gluteal injections, trauma, or cellulite. These irregularities are treated simultaneously in the manner described later.

SURGICAL TECHNIQUE
Anesthesia and Preparation

The presence of an anesthesiologist during the surgical procedure when using intravenous (IV) sedation or in other kinds of anesthesia is imperative to maintain patients and the monitoring of the vital signs and safety. When Illouz[1] described the liposuction technique in 1980, most of the procedures needed to be done with epidural or general anesthesia. In 1987, Klein[7] introduced the tumescent anesthesia technique, a formula that allowed the surgeon to inject local anesthesia in many different large areas of the body with a small dose of the lidocaine, adrenaline, and saline solution at room temperature; this could be done with or without sedation. In 1989, I altered Klein's formula, increasing the concentration of lidocaine and adrenaline and changing the saline solution to Ringer lactate.[8]

Toledo local infiltration solution is as follows: 20 mL 2% lidocaine, 1 mL adrenaline, 500 mL Ringer lactate, and 5 mL 3% sodium bicarbonate. The proportion of infiltration in relation to the aspirated solution should be between1:1 and 1.5:1. I inject 1 mL of fluid per 1 mL of fat that I estimate to aspirate. This proportion avoids pulmonary edema and lidocaine overdose. For body contour, I prefer IV sedation or general anesthesia with midazolam, fentanyl, and propofol. Maintenance is done with propofol 0.025 mg/kg/min and fentanyl 50 μg slowly. Before injecting the local anesthesia solution, I warm it to 37°C because hypothermia alters the coagulation factors, increasing bleeding, and it can cause coagulopathy. By heating every IV and subcutaneous fluid

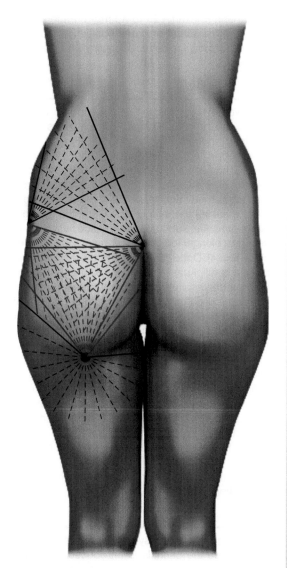

Fig. 2. With these three incisions, one in the trochanter, one in the inter-gluteal fold and one in the sub-gluteal fold, we can treat the buttocks, flanks, lateral and posterior thighs. In black are the areas of fat aspiration, and in red of fat injection.

to 37°C, I reduce hypothermia and postoperative shivering.[9] Forced air warming (with hot air blankets) prevents hypothermia and avoids metabolic and blood composition changes, which leads to complications like infections, blood loss, heart attacks, and even death. I know that long procedures increase the risk of complications. I try not to exceed 3 hours of surgery. Procedures that are longer than 2 hours with patients in the same position require the use of compression boots to prevent deep vein thrombosis (DVT). Drug prevention of DVT can be done with nadroparin calcium (Fraxieparine) (7500 UI/d) or enoxaparin (Clexane) 20 to 40 mg/d. Patients are treated in the lateral or prone position, according to the problem, for better access to the areas to be treated.

Instruments

My favorite tools are the 60-mL Toomey tip syringes and zirconium-fused Tulip cannulas (Tulip Medical Products, San Diego, CA) (**Fig. 3**). They slide better and are especially good for fibrotic areas. The cannula fits better to the syringe body and not only at the tip. It gives a much firmer grip than the catheter tip syringes, without the possibility of breaking the syringe tip. Once the cannula penetrates the subcutaneous tissue, vacuum is kept by a plunger lock in the shape of a U or horseshoe (**Fig. 4**). Once I have aspirated the fat and the syringe is full, I pass the syringe to the nurse who will treat the aspirated fat for possible reinjection. The nurse decants the syringes and takes note of the amount of total aspirated fluid and pure fat from each syringe, which is done for each area treated. I finish the surgery with a map with the exact amounts of aspirated and injected fat. I use special cannulas for fibrotic areas, areas of difficult aspiration, and secondary procedures. For treating skin irregularities, cellulite depressions, or liposuction sequelae, I use a special 3-mm-gauge V-tip cannula dissector, 20 to 35 cm long, adapted to the 60-mL syringe. It can dissect, suction, or inject fat where necessary. It is an important element for treating certain iatrogenic liposuction defects (**Fig. 5**).

Fat Aspiration

Aspirating fat with the syringe is very straightforward. Once the cannula is introduced, I pull the

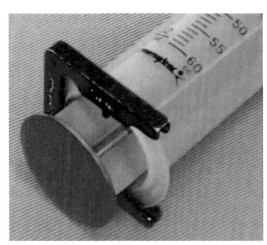

Fig. 4. The 60-cc Toomey tip syringes connect to the zirconium fused Tulip cannulas. The cannula fits better to the syringe body and not only at the tip. Once the cannula penetrates the subcutaneous tissue vacuum is kept by a plunger lock in the shape of a U or horseshoe.

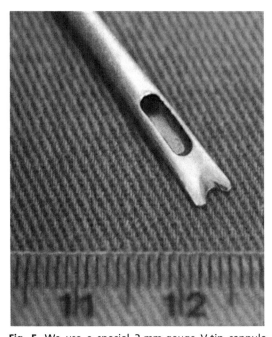

Fig. 5. We use a special 3-mm-gauge V-tip cannula dissector, 20-35 cm long, adapted to the 60-cc syringe for treating skin irregularities, cellulite depressions, or liposuction sequaelae. It can dissect, suction, or inject fat where necessary. It is an important element for treating certain iatrogenic liposuction defects.

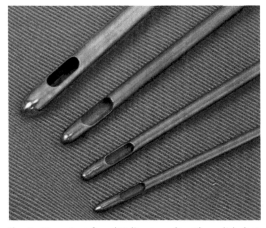

Fig. 3. Zirconium fused Tulip cannulas. They slide better and cause less damage to the fat cells.

plunger and lock it, creating vacuum in the syringe. With gentle in-and-out movements in a fan shape, I aspirate all the areas that need treatment. I aspirate fat from the back, axilla, flanks, abdomen, and thighs. Sometimes fat also has to be aspirated from the lower third of the buttock. Superficial liposuction in this area will create some skin retraction, which, combined with fat injection of the upper part, creates the appearance of a lifted buttock. I check skin regularity by wetting the area to facilitate visualizing depressions or bulges. Once I have enough fat, it is decanted or centrifuged and immediately reinjected.

Fat Injection

Harvesting, cleaning, and injecting fat is a procedure that should be followed precisely in order to obtain good results. Excessive manipulation of the harvested fat must be avoided. I do not sieve or expose fat cells to air to avoid trauma and oxidation. The syringes with fat are centrifuged at 1500 rpm for 1 minute or decanted for 10 minutes. The anesthetic fluid is separated from the fat cells, and the pure fat is gently injected. The fat graft's ability to obtain nutrition through plasmatic imbibition occurs approximately 1.5 mm from the vascularized edge. I can inject up to 500 mL of fat on each buttock, injected in parallel threads subcutaneously, leaving space for neovascularization. I use 3 different incisions to avoid the formation of lakes of fat, instead injecting threads of fat that should be no thicker than 3 mm. Fat is injected in the subcutaneous,

subdermal and intramuscular areas (**Fig. 6**). If patients want more volume than I can obtain with 500 mL on each side, I suggest a second procedure after 3 to 6 months (**Figs. 7–9**).

Recently I have started using stem cell–based therapies for buttock augmentation. If I am going to use adipose-derived stem cells (ADSCs), 60 mL of fat is harvested 10 days before the procedure in the office under local anesthesia. This amount is sent to the laboratory[10] for adipose stem cells (ASC) isolation and ex vivo expansion. I can obtain around 500 million ADSCs with one amplification, to be mixed with 1000 mL of fat. The system is fast; it requires 10 days of cell culture, without the use of synthetic scaffold. It is safe because more than 1000 patients in clinical trials have received mesenchymal stem cells, and no adverse events have been reported. On the day of the procedure, I enrich the fat to be injected with the previously prepared ADSC.

Postoperative care is as follows: Patients will leave the operating room and go to the recovery room for about 1 hour, already wearing the corset and the DVT-prevention stockings. I prefer my patients to spend the first night in the clinic because the peak of the lidocaine absorption happens around 12 hours after the injection. Another reason is that nurses can help patients to ambulate early and give medications. The next morning, patients will have a shower; the dressing and corset will be changed; and they will be discharged. After 2 days they can walk a mile. Antibiotics are prescribed for 5 to 7 days. There can be temporary mild pain, especially in the first 48 hours, which

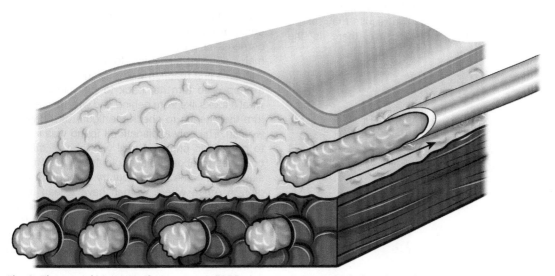

Fig. 6. The cannula injecting fat in retrograde movements, in 3 mm thick threads, in three areas (layers) sub-cutaneously, into the fat layer and into the muscle.

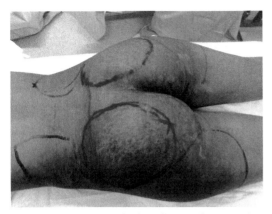

Fig. 7. Patients are marked in the standing position. On the operating table, the deformities change shape. I mark the areas to be suctioned in blue and the areas to be augmented in red.

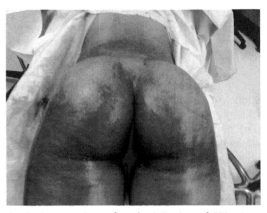

Fig. 9. Same patient after the injection of 500 mL on each buttock.

can be treated with analgesics. Swelling, soreness, numbness, and bruising usually last a few weeks. Dressings are applied on the small incisions. There will be a leak of the anesthetic fluid through the incisions in the first 24 hours. Dressings will be changed daily. Showering is allowed after 24 hours but no immersion bath. The girdle should be worn for 3 to 4 weeks. Stitches will be removed between the fifth and seventh day. Driving and lying on the back is allowed after a week. There is no problem with sitting straight because I do not usually inject fat in the ischial area. Patients can go back to work in 2 to 3 weeks and can exercise and sunbathe in 4 to 6 weeks or more, depending on the bruising. Fading and flattening of the small scars can take between 3 months and 2 years.

Liposculpture improves body contour and increases self-confidence. The results may take a few months to show because there is the possibility of fluid retention following surgery with prolonged swelling. Occasionally, a secondary procedure or touch-up may be indicated to improve certain areas, most times under local anesthesia. A special massage, called *manual lymphatic drainage*, helps with the swelling and bruising in the postoperative period, increasing comfort. If the weight remains the same, the results should be permanent, especially when combined with diet and exercise.

DISCUSSION

The need for buttock augmentation came because Brazilians at the time preferred smaller breasts and bigger buttocks, a body type different to the North American and European standards. Today the Brazilian woman also prefer bigger breasts; but in the 1980s, running and exercising had become fashionable and bodies were more athletic. The origin of this fixation of Brazilians with women's derrières is unknown. I have read the work of many sociologists trying to understand why a woman's first reaction when trying a new outfit in a shop is to turn her back to the mirror to see what it looks like from behind and why men always turn their heads to check the figure of a passing woman. The only explanation I found was related to our ethnic origins. Brazil was one of the last countries to abolish slavery in 1888. Most of the slaves that came to the country came from a region in Africa where women have a lean upper body and heavy buttocks and thighs, the so-called gynoid type of body. The mixture of the Portuguese colonizers with the Africans created a type of body with mostly fine waists and round buttocks.

In 2005, I moved to Dubai to start my practice in the United Arab Emirates. Dubai is now becoming

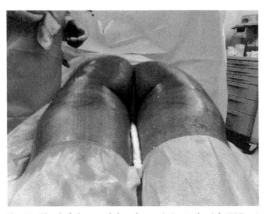

Fig. 8. The left buttock has been injected with 500 mL of fat. The difference from the right side is visible.

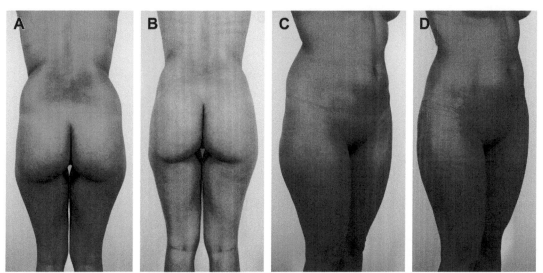

Fig. 10. (*A–D*) A 28-year-old Moroccan patient before and 1 year after liposculpture of flanks and thighs, with augmentation of trochanter and buttocks.

a hub for medical tourism; in my practice, most of the patients are still local Emiratis, at 40%. The other 60% are divided between patients of more than 73 different nationalities, some of them expats living in the city and others traveling here only for medical tourism. One can imagine the complexity in pleasing patients with so many different concepts of beauty. In Dubai, buttock augmentation has become more popular during the last decade and is one of the top 10 procedures I perform every year (**Figs. 10–14**). Complications are rare. I had 3 cases of infection by staphylococcus epidermidis that were cured with antibiotics. I also had one case of seroma, which had to be drained.

After many years of injecting purified fat, I started using stem cell–based therapies for buttock augmentation. My experience is still not long enough to judge if my results will match the literature. Regenerative medicine using autologous adipose tissue is an emerging field in plastic surgery, and I am using the method to increase graft viability. Studies show that a triple-blind placebo-controlled trial comparing the survival of fat grafts enriched with ADSC versus nonenriched fat grafts had significantly higher residual volumes: 80.9% versus 16.3% of the initial volumes of injected fat. I hope to be able to improve the reabsorption rate of my results. I still face some problems using ADSC either because patients do not want to

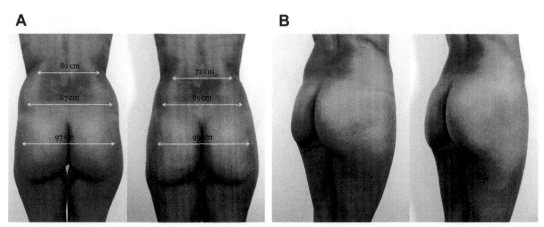

Fig. 11. (*A, B*) A 35-year-old patient before and 6 months after liposculpture of the flanks, lateral thighs, and buttocks, showing a 2-cm increase in the buttock circumference, even with a weight reduction of 5 kg.

A   **B**

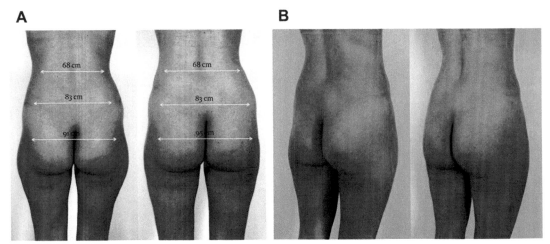

Fig. 12. (*A, B*) A 42-year-old patient before and 1 year after aspiration of fat from the lateral thighs and injection of 420 mL into each buttock.

A   **B**

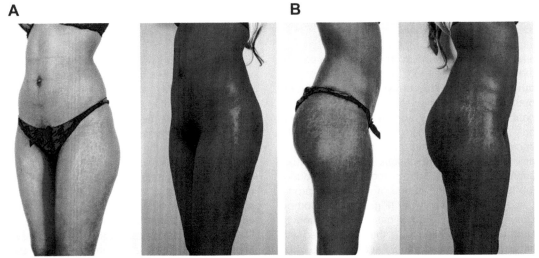

Fig. 13. (*A, B*) A 23-year-old African model (the patient on **Figs. 4–6**) before and 1 year after aspiration of fat from the flanks, abdomen, and lateral thighs with injection in the buttocks.

A   **B**

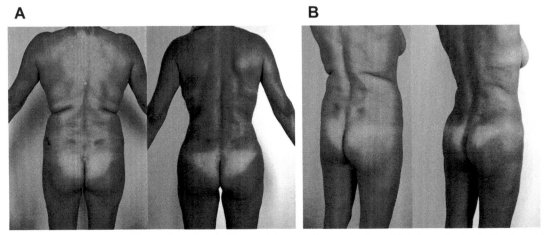

Fig. 14. (*A, B*) A 45-year-old French patient before and 1 year after aspiration of fat from the back, flanks, and abdomen and fat grafting of the buttocks.

wait the 2 or 3 weeks between the procedures or because of the significant cost increase.

SUMMARY

Buttock augmentation with fat grafting has become one of the most sought after procedures in plastic surgery. The technique can be done with standard instruments; but to achieve good results, there are certain specifications that need to be strictly followed (ie, the technique for fat harvesting, treatment, and injection). Recently tissue-engineering techniques have been introduced with the hope of increasing the fat graft survival. It is still unclear if the increase in cost and time will eventually justify the use of ADSC. Some patients who want bigger buttocks are difficult to please. I always explain that there is a limit to the amount of fat that can be injected in one procedure. Usually I inject 500 mL per side on a normal patient and 600 mL on a bigger patient, maximum. With more than this amount, I start injecting lakes of fat, which will suffer necrosis and will be absorbed. Fat necrosis is usually absorbed without the need of any intervention. Seromas are rare; but if they happen, they are aspirated. A postoperative control computed tomography scan can confirm the need for aspiration. Patients who do not like the partial reabsorption of the fat are informed they will need a second procedure. Preoperative photographs, weight, and measurements are vital records in these procedures. I always inform patients that the reabsorption will be around 50%. I hope to improve the fat survival with the new ADSC technique.

REFERENCES

1. Illouz YG. A new method for localized lipodystrophies. Rev Chir Esthet 1980;4(6):19.
2. Fournier P. Liposculpture - Ma technique. Paris: Arnette; 1989.
3. Matsudo PK, Toledo LS. Experience of injected fat grafting. Aesthetic Plast Surg 1988;12:35–8.
4. Peer LA. Loss of weight and volume in human fat grafts: with postulation of a cell survival theory. Plast Reconstr Surg 1950;5:217–30.
5. Toledo LS. Syringe aspiration liposculpture, Teleplast. ASPRS/PSEF; 1995.
6. Toledo LS. Syringe liposculpture. Clin Plast Surg 1996;23(4):683–93.
7. Klein JA. The tumescent technique for liposuction surgery. Am J Cosmetic Surg 1987;4:263–7.
8. Toledo LS. Superficial syringe liposculpture. Annals of the International Symposium Recent Advances in Plastic Surgery. São Paulo, Brazil, March 3–5, 1990. p. 446.
9. Toledo LS, Carneiro JD, Regatieri FL. The effect of hypothermia on coagulation and its implications for infiltration in lipoplasty: a review. Aesthet Surg J 2001;21(1):40–4.
10. Bioscience Clinic – Middle East FZ-LLC - Al Razi Building 64-Dubai Health Care City, Dubai UAE.

Fat Grafting for Treatment of Burns, Burn Scars, and Other Difficult Wounds

Nelson Sarto Piccolo, MD[a],*, Mônica Sarto Piccolo, MD, MSc[b],
Maria Thereza Sarto Piccolo, MD, PhD[b]

KEYWORDS

- Fat grafting • Burns • Wounds • Burn scars • Burn sequelae • Wound healing • Scar remodeling

KEY POINTS

- The use of fat grafting has changed our practice dramatically, mainly in relation to our previous routines of using immediate excision and grafting in burns of the hands and in relation to our early (practically the immediate day after admission) use of muscle flaps for exposed bone fractures in patients who were traditionally referred (6–8 weeks after the original injury) from a local state hospital with subacute wounds and open fractures of the middle or lower third of the leg.
- Fat grafting has also greatly influenced the way we treat hypertrophic scars as a consequence of burn wounds.
- One of the most pleasant surprises in using fat grafts is the minimal incidence (or none) of hypertrophic scarring on the healing of wounds treated with one or more sessions of fat grafting.

 The Authors present three videos of procedures: Video 1 presents chronic wound debridement and fat injections for skin grafting. Video 2 presents fat injection under finger burn wounds. Video 3 presents fat injections under a facial scar. These videos can be viewed at www.plasticsurgery.theclinics.com/

OVERVIEW

Fat grafting has been used worldwide taking advantage of the benefits of adipose-derived stem cells (ADSC's) for regenerative purposes and their ability to differentiate in fat, bone, cartilage, muscle, and possibly other tissues. They also have a great variety of regenerative and metabolic properties, and growth factors (eg, epidermal growth factor, transforming growth factor-β, hepatocyte growth factor, platelet-derived growth factor, basic fibroblast growth factor). Fat on the lipoaspirate can be isolated and/or treated by physical or chemical methods, in the operating room, or in a laboratory setup.[1–8]

Burns and Wound Healing

The most typical burn that occurs in a child in our area of the world is a burn caused by hot liquids during preparation or consumption of a meal, followed by sudden flame of ethanol, used by the child or in the vicinity of an adult using ethanol.

[a] Division of Plastic Surgery, Pronto Socorro para Queimaduras, Rua 5, n. 439 - Setor Oeste, Goiânia, Goiás 74115 060, Brazil; [b] Pronto Socorro para Queimaduras, Rua 5, n. 439 - Setor Oeste, Goiânia, Goiás 74115 060, Brazil
* Corresponding author.
E-mail address: nelsonpiccolo@yahoo.com

Clin Plastic Surg 42 (2015) 263–283
http://dx.doi.org/10.1016/j.cps.2014.12.009

In the adult population, most commonly burns are caused by ethanol, a work-related injury (electrical, hot surfaces, plastic extrusion/packaging machine, and so forth), or a motorcycle accident (contact burns with the exhaust system, or friction burn/fracture in a fall).

Because our burn service was founded in 1968, and it is open to all patients regardless of payment or insurance, in the past 46 years we have seen more than 320,000 burn cases. Thus, we have slowly evolved to become a burn and wound care center, receiving a substantial number of patients with subacute or chronic wounds, either in consequence of a motorcycle or motor vehicle accident, or related to vascular insufficiency or diabetes.

Patients who are candidates for fat grafting procedure at our service are those with (1) hypertrophic scars that are not improving or not being controlled by pressure garments at 6 or more weeks after healing, (2) burn wounds at 3 weeks or more with no apparent progression to healing, (3) subacute burn wounds or other wounds transferred to us within more than 6 weeks after the accident or wound, and (4) venous or diabetic ulcers.

Surgical Approach

In wounds, we use the Coleman technique, repeating injections (and reharvesting) every 2 to 4 weeks until healing or until a definite procedure (eg, wound closure, skin grafting, flap, or other) is performed. After healing, injections under the scar are performed at 3-month intervals, also via the Coleman technique.[9-12] This approach is also taken with patients with scars who seek our service for consultation after being treated elsewhere.

TREATMENT GOALS AND PLANNED OUTCOMES

The use of fat grafting as an adjuvant treatment in acute and subacute burn wounds and in chronic vascular wounds (venous insufficiency or diabetic arterial disease) takes advantage of fat's benefits: a variety of metabolic and regenerative properties, increasing vascularization, and enhancing the tissue regeneration process. When these wounds are treated with repeated fat grafting (15–21 days apart), healing is the planned outcome.[13-15]

When treating burn scars, the objective is to decrease the amount of hypertrophy (fibrosis), diminishing the scar thickness and increasing scar malleability. We also use this technique to decrease fibrosis around bone joints and at releasing tendon adhesions.[16-19]

PREOPERATIVE PLANNING AND PREPARATION

Patients with subacute burn wounds (more than 3 weeks in our Service without apparent progression to healing), open fractures of the tibia, associated to nonhealing or poorly healing wounds, chronic venous insufficiency, or diabetic arterial disease wounds are selected for adjuvant treatment with fat injection. In open wounds, injections are performed under general anesthesia, in 15- to 21-day intervals.

Patients with hypertrophic scarring after healing of a burn or keloids of any origin are also selected for treatment with fat injection. Repeat injections (up to four injections total) are performed at 8- to 12-week intervals.

Donor areas are "rotated" as needed and fat most frequently is obtained from the abdomen, thighs, or lateral upper buttocks. When necessary, shaving of the pubic area or proximal thigh is performed in the operating room, immediately before the procedure. Puncture incisions for introduction of the liposuction cannula are placed on the midline, at the suprapubic crease; medial to the femoral pulse, at the inguinal crease; or in the middle axillary line, at the upper border of the iliac bone.

The actual volume of harvested lipoaspirate should be at least twice the anticipated volume planned to be injected, and at least four times this volume if one is also planning to have fat deposited over the wound.

PATIENT POSITIONING

Patients are supine when using the abdomen or thighs as donor areas or on lateral decubitus when obtaining fat from the lateral upper thighs. Fat is usually injected while the patient is supine.

PROCEDURAL APPROACH

Fat harvesting and fat injection are sterile surgical procedures and should be performed only in accredited operation rooms under rigorous, completely sterile technique. In patients with scars (healed wounds), the donor area and recipient area are individually prepared and draped in the usual manner. In patients with open, nonhealed wounds, the recipient area is prepared only after the planned amount of fat is obtained, while it is being centrifuged and distributed in various syringes.

Fat is harvested from the patient himself or herself, using a 10-mL Luer Lok syringe, attached to a 3-mm cannula, with two 3-mm side openings distally, with 10-, 15-, or 20-cm length, according to the harvesting site. In children weighing less than 25 kg, we prefer 20-mL syringes and multi (micro) perforated cannulas, which enforce a higher negative pressure ensuring more even and efficient fat harvesting, respectively. Occasionally, in very small patients (our smallest patient weighted 13 kg), it may be necessary to harvest fat from more than one donor site.

One or more distally plugged 10-mL syringes containing the obtained fat is centrifuged at 3000 rpm for 3 minutes on a 30-degree angle centrifuge. The obtained compound has a top layer of oil, a middle layer of fat (with the stromal vascular fraction (SVF) within at its lower portion), and an aqueous inferior layer. The top layer of oil is discarded while the plug still is on the syringe. The plug is then removed and the aqueous layer drains out per gravity. The remaining compound is sequentially injected into "insulin" syringes without the plunger, which is then replaced (**Fig. 1**).

Using a 16-gauge needle, a perforation is made at an acute angle in healthy skin in the periphery of the wound or the scar. A 1.8-mm outside diameter (1.2-mm internal diameter) 70-mm long cannula already connected to the 1-mL syringe is inserted through the needle puncture hole and (forcefully) driven immediately under the wound bed or the scar. Fat is then deposited in a retrograde manner, in several "passes" until the entire area is injected (via as many puncture sites as needed around the periphery of the scar or wound). On average, 1.6 to 2.0 mL is injected per each 10 cm^2 area and it is necessary to make 25 to 30 passes to inject 1 mL. In chronic wounds, the induration, "healed" area in the periphery of the remaining wound, is also injected (**Figs. 2** and **3**, Videos 1–3).

Occasionally, when there are fracture lines of bone loss "voids" or exposed bone, fat is injected through the wound (**Fig. 4**A). Also, in wounds where the entire thickness of the skin or more tissue has been lost, fat is also deposited in a zigzag manner over the entire surface of the wound, also using the same cannula as for the injection (see **Fig. 4**B).

There are patients with lesions that have been partially or poorly treated, sometimes who did not even have appropriate debridement of their original (or consequential) wound. In these cases,

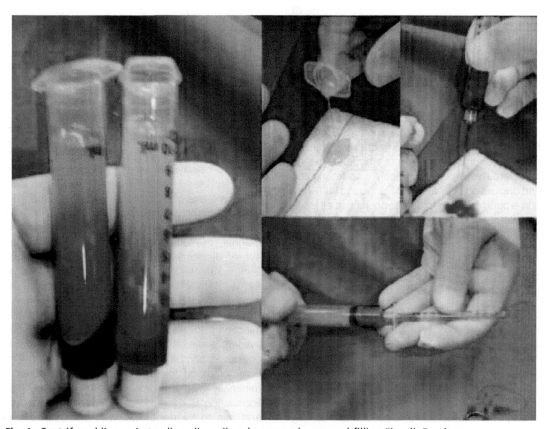

Fig. 1. Centrifuged lipoaspirate, discarding oil and aqueous layers, and filling "insulin" syringe.

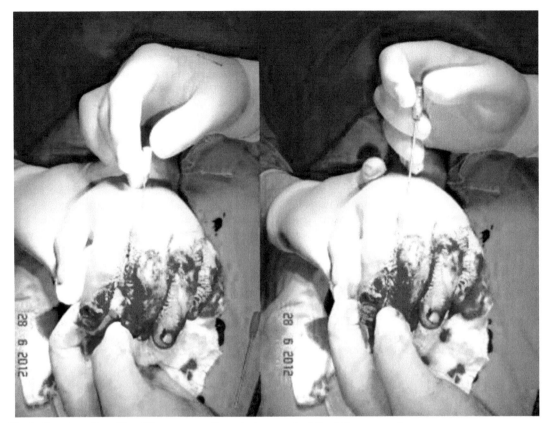

Fig. 2. Puncture site with a 16-gauge needle and placement of the 1.8-mm canulla.

we perform one or more debridements, complementing them, if necessary, immediately before fat injection. In cases of open fractures, regardless of the presence or absence of internal or external hardware, we proceed routinely with fat injection and deposition in all areas of the wound with injection around and under, and deposition in all loss of substance voids, including bone spaces (please see Video 1).

POTENTIAL COMPLICATIONS AND THEIR MANAGEMENT
Infection

Although infection is a common complication in burn and other trauma wounds, we have experienced no complications related to infection, even with injections through burn and other wounds and with fat deposited over the wound. We recommend, however, in wounds that are heavily contaminated, a debridement 2 days before the fat injection procedure.

Fat Grafting Technique or Procedure

Complications in fat grafting may be related to the procedure or technique themselves, mostly because of physical trauma to underlying structures by the cannula or other injection device. We favor the use of blunt cannulas with distal side openings, connected to a small-volume (1 mL) syringe, and that fat be injected in a retrograde manner, in multiple passes, depositing multiple, evenly distributed, streaks of fat with less than 2-mm diameter. When injecting under thick scar tissue, it may be safer to previously pass the cannula under the scar in several directions, "opening" the way for faster movements while injecting fat. This may be particularly useful when treating areas on the neck and face, where noble structures can be easily injured or perforated.[19,20]

Although fat injection could be considered a minimally invasive procedure, fat obtention by liposuction is considered an invasive procedure and has to be performed with extreme caution and technical rigor, if such complications as

A

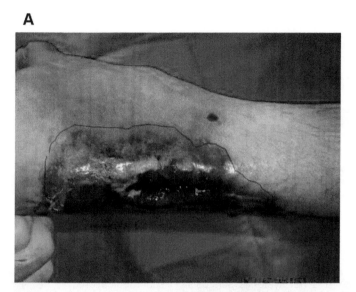

B

Fig. 3. (*A*) A 46-year-old patient with diabetes with 4.5-month Achilles tendon wound (patient does not extend foot). Drawing indicates area to be injected. (*B*) Cannula position indicates direction of injection on the previously planned area (*top*); puncture with 16-gauge needle (*bottom left*) and injection being performed also under the recently healed area (*bottom right*).

C

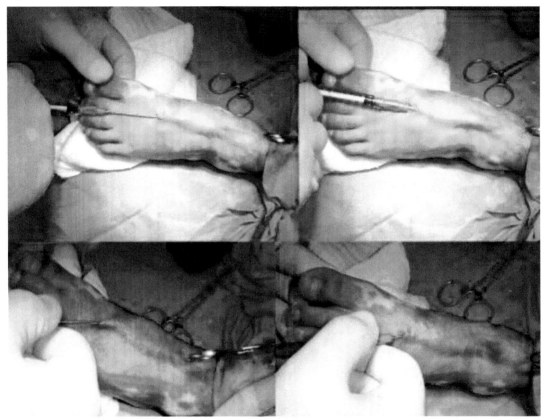

Fig. 3. (*continued*). (*C*) Fat is deposited in all directions and multiple sites until the entire planned area is injected.

asymmetry and trauma to fascia, to muscle, or even to viscera are to be avoided.

Because fat acquisition from very small patients is still infrequent, we recommend extreme care in harvesting it, while endeavoring to be symmetric and to obtain deeper fat (under Scarpa fascia) to avoid the occurrence of future superficial irregularities. Also, using slightly higher negative pressure (20-mL syringe) and multi (micro) perforated cannulas ensures faster and more precise fat harvesting. Assurance of long-term follow-up visits must be provided as the small patient grows.

Subdermal or Deep Vessel Injury

In the rare case that a subdermal or deeper vessel may be injured, local pressure and abortion of the injection on that site should be the immediate action. Ensuing ecchymosis disappears with time and the patient must be reassured about the evolution of this most unusual complication.

Edema

In scar cases, postoperative edema is a frequent event in the immediate days after the procedure and the patient must be warned about it.

Venous Ulcers

In patients with venous ulcer, postural drainage is fundamental for the success of treatment and one should inform the patient that the improvement of the wound does not substitute postural measures (**Fig. 5**). In diabetic arterial disease, adequate footwear and proper foot care is a must for progressive weight bearing after healing without recurrence (**Fig. 6**).

POSTPROCEDURAL CARE

In wounds, a closed dressing is applied with a first layer of petroleum jelly gauze, followed by several layers of fine mesh gauze that are soaked with double-strength Dakin solution

A

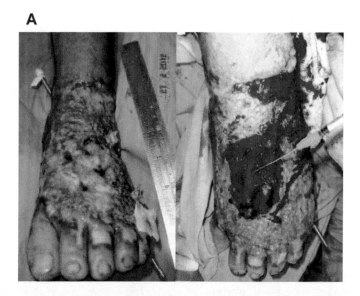

B

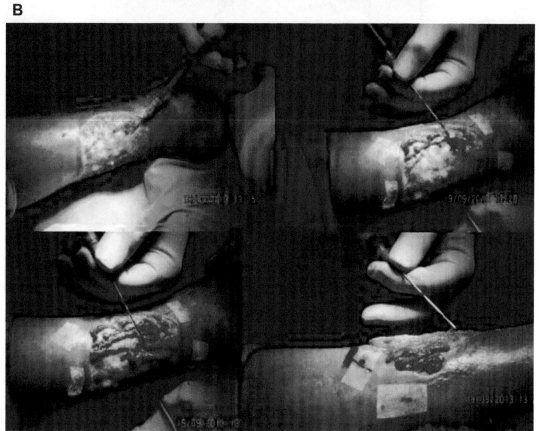

Fig. 4. (*A*) A 32-year-old patient 15 days after grafting with central loss debridement (*left*) and at injection through the wound (*right*). (*B*) A 62-year-old woman with diabetes with 7.5-year-old wound, being injected through the wound (*top left*); and also having fat deposited over the wound (note paper tape dressing previous punctures sites).

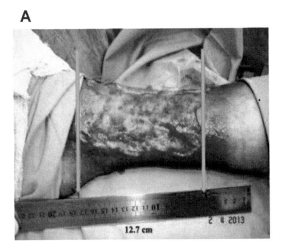

Fig. 5. (*A*) A 68-year-old patient with Chagas disease with 8-year-old venous ulcer (2 days after debridement). (*B*) Evolution of the wound after two injections in 27 days (*top left*); successful skin grafting (*top right*) and take (*bottom left*); and eventual loss (*bottom right*), after missing three dressings (patient was admitted for megacolon surgery elsewhere). Although there was a skin graft loss, the wound remained contracted about 30% compared with the original size.

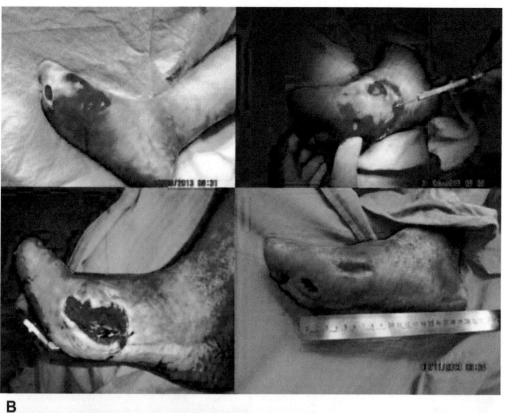

Fig. 6. (*A*) A 71-year-old patient with diabetes with 2-year-old wound, which was injected with fat and debrided, progressively improving over an 8-week period. (*B*) After second injection (*top left*), medial foot evolved to cure (*top right*), and despite improvement (*bottom left*), persistent weight bearing without shoes led to recurrence of plantar wound (medial wound remained healed) (*bottom right*).

(Henry Drysdale Dakin, 1880–1952, English chemist). A bandage finishes the dressing. Dressings are changed every 2 days. In scars, a piece of paper tape is placed on the puncture sites (**Fig. 7**).

REHABILITATION AND RECOVERY

During treatment, patients are followed by the entire dedicated team. Support from all related paramedical specialties is constantly provided. In most of the burn sequelae cases, fat grafting is used as a measure to bring relief in scar hypertrophy and

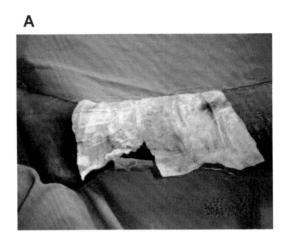

Fig. 7. (*A*) Appearance of the petroleum jelly gauze in a 2-day-old dressing. Note that there are no secretions and one can see the yellow surviving fat through the gauze (same patient in **Fig. 17**). (*B*) Progressive appearance of the surface deposited fat, which survives and slowly turns into healthy granulation tissue (same patient in **Fig. 17**).

restriction. It has proved to be very efficient, occasionally avoiding and frequently postponing scar removal reconstructive procedures.

As part of their rehabilitation and our goal to attain full patient recovery, reconstructive procedures aiming at partial or complete scar removal are usually offered at the time of scar maturation. Our main method of reconstruction is the use of superposed tissue expanders, either forming an L-, J-, or V-shaped composition, matching part of or the entire desired removal area. Sequential procedures are indicated as needed.

OUTCOMES

All 240 patients with burn or trauma wounds treated with this technique healed. Of the 42 patients with venous or diabetic ulcers, 40 healed. The two unhealed patients were a 68-year-old woman with an 8-year-old venous ulcer on the right leg who lost the skin graft 15 days after the procedure while at another institution (she had two successful injections, which led to a initially successful skin grafting; see **Fig. 5**); and, a 72-year-old man with diabetes with one wound in the plantar area and another wound in the medial distal foot, who had a recurrence of the plantar wound after noncompliance with temporary no weight bearing recommendations (see **Fig. 6**).

All 87 patients with scars treated with this technique related improvement, which was also noticeable after each injection, except for one teenager with facial scars in whom although no visible improvement was noticed after the first injection, but who related great improvement in suppleness of the scar. Subsequent injections demonstrated visible improvements (**Figs. 8–12**).

In complex burn or trauma wounds, patients were treated with fat injection fostering wound healing, and during the posthealing phase, favoring periarticular fibrosis improvement and bone formation (**Figs. 13–17**).

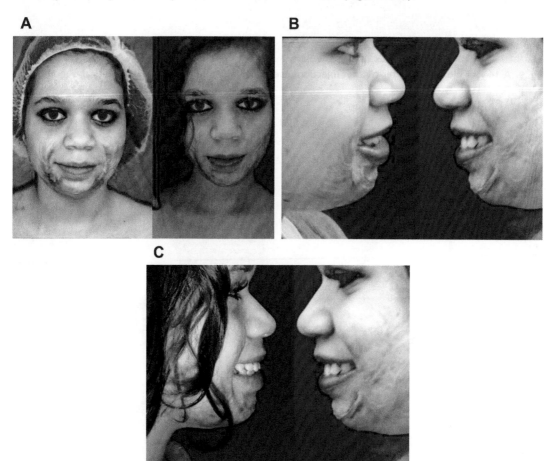

Fig. 8. (*A*) A 14-year-old patient with two injections on her left side and Z-plasty plus one injection on her right side. (*B*) Same patient, after injection on her left side. Note smile showing three teeth on left (injected with fat), two teeth on right (Z-plasty). (*C*) Same patient, after two injections on left and one injection on right side. Note similar smiles indicating similar suppleness of scar on perioral area.

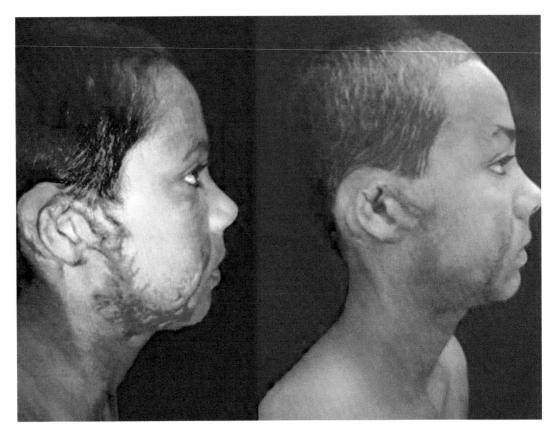

Fig. 9. A 14-year-old patient after two fat injections every 2 months under facial scar. Results at 5 months.

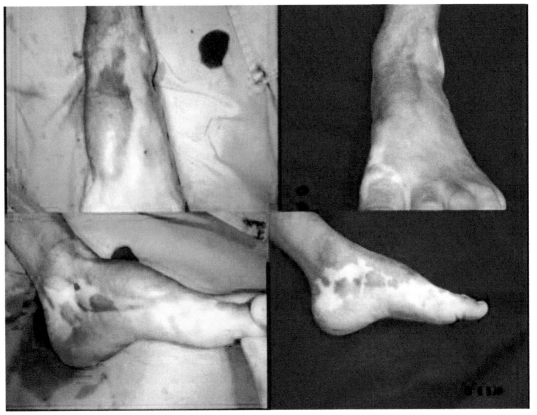

Fig. 10. A 4-year-old patient 5 months after three injections (first injection patient weighted 13 kg, at third injection 19 kg). Note complete remission of hypertrophic scar volume.

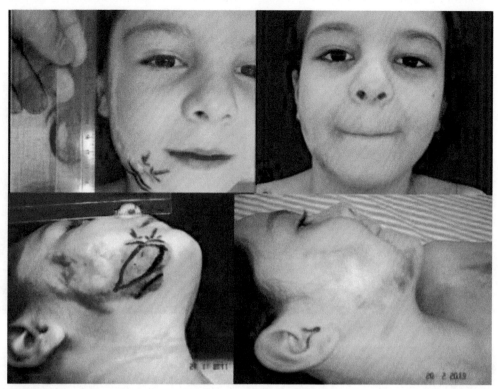

Fig. 11. A 6-year-old patient treated with two fat injections at 3-month intervals and initial partial resection of scar (ellipsis drawn on scar). Result at 8 months on *top* and *bottom right*.

A

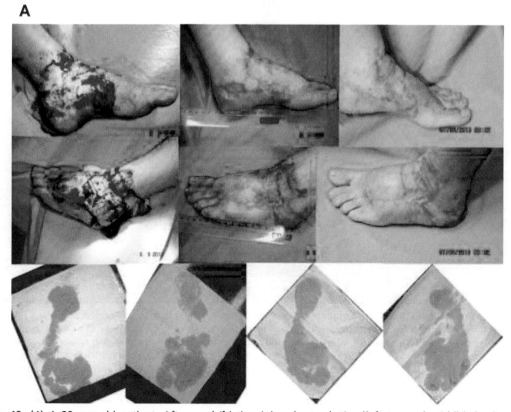

Fig. 12. (*A*) A 38-year-old patient. After crush/friction injury by truck tire (*left top* and *middle*); healing at 3 months with two fat injections and skin grafting (*center top* and *middle*); 8 months posthealing with three more injections under the scar and around joint spaces, dramatically improving appearance and function (*right top* and *middle*). Note plantar impression at healing time (*left bottom*) and at 8 months postcure (*right bottom*).

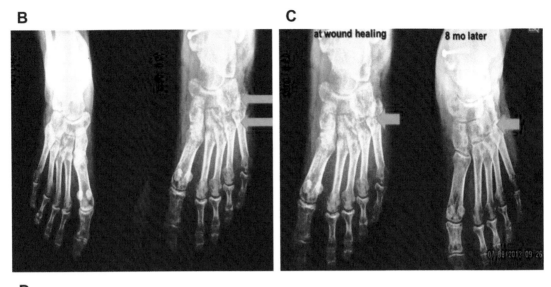

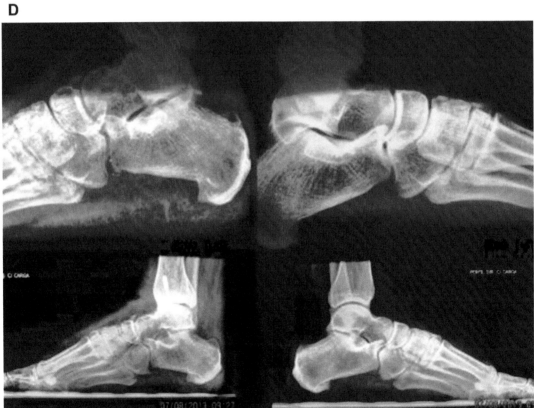

Fig. 12. (continued). (B) Right and left feet. *Arrow* shows blurring of the joint spaces on left at healing time. (C) Left foot. Note evolution from joint spaces "blurring" on radiograph (fibrosis) at the time of healing to normalcy 8 months posthealing after three fat injections around joint spaces and under the scar. *Left arrow* shows blurring of joint spaces, *right arrow* shows improvement with "clearing" of the joint spaces. (D) Same patient, showing left foot longitudinal arch higher at healing time (*top left*) and normal (*bottom left*) after three fat injections around the joint spaces and under the residual scar.

A

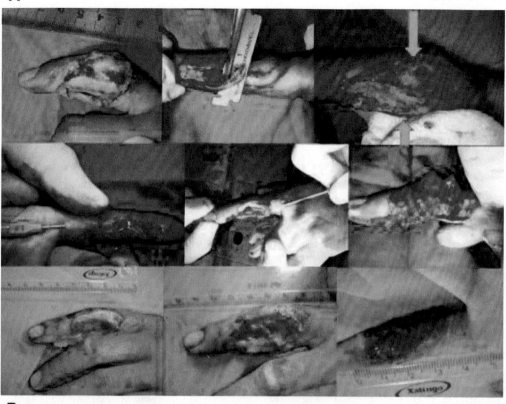

B

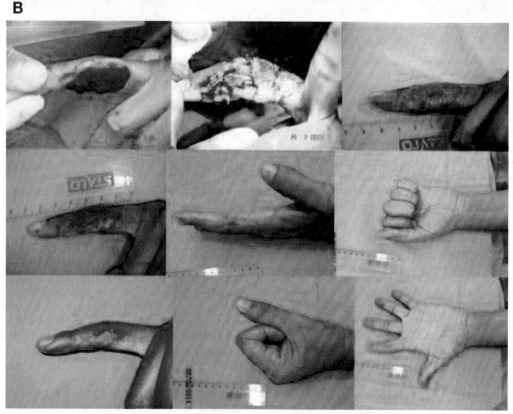

Fig. 13. (*A*) A 32-year-old victim of 330-V discharge; debridement exposing deep structures (neurovascular bundle plus tendon; *top*); fat injection under the wound and fat deposited on the wound (*middle*); evolution in 1 (*bottom left*), 4 (*bottom center*), and 9 (*bottom right*) days. *Top arrow* shows tendon band and *lower arrow* shows microvascular bundle. (*B*) Skin grafting at 13 days (*top left* and *center*); 12 days after grafting (*top right*), healing at 28 days (15 days after grafting; *middle left*); appearance and range of motion at 14 months postcure. No hypertrophy, no adhesions.

A

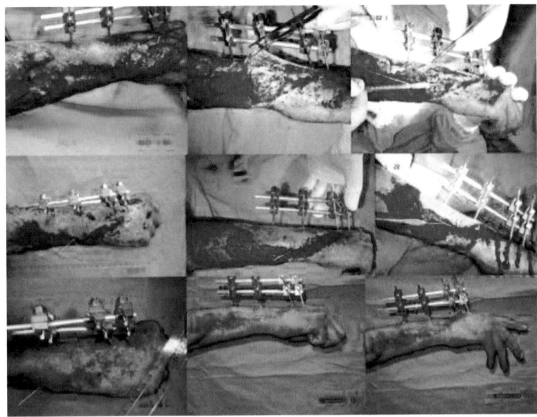

Fig. 14. (*A*) A 28-year-old patient 10 days after motorcycle accident plus distal ulnar fracture (*top left*); initial debridement (suture of III, IV, and V ruptured extensor tendons) (*top center*) and fat injection (*top right*) at 4 days (*middle left*) at 10 days (*middle center*) followed by a second injection 15 days later (*middle right*), healing at 33 days (*bottom left*). Results at 3 months, no hypertrophy (*bottom center* and *right*).

In the past 3 years, we progressively changed our previous routine of debridement and practically immediate muscle flap covered with a skin graft for open fracture wounds on the leg, to a routine of sequential fat grafting, either creating a healthy bed for a future skin graft, or allowing it to evolve to complete healing.

CLINICAL RESULTS IN THE LITERATURE

Several studies indicate that the SVF within the collected fat is richer in ADSC's, and some have warranted that the enrichment of fat grafting with cells from the SVF equals cell-assisted lipotransfer. Although there are apparent advantages in doing that, we believe that there are enough stem cells on the centrifuged fat to warrant the obvious benefits we have noticed on our patients who were treated with the Coleman technique.[21–25]

Enriching fat grafting with platelet-rich plasma or platelet-rich fibrin may also become additional alternatives to perpetrate and to improve results. These authors state that there could be even a higher or more significant load of growth factors in these additional compounds.[26,27]

Fat injection to improve healing in different types of wounds is most likely caused by several factors in the adipose-derived stem cells themselves and by the growth factors already present in the injected fat, contributing to diminish fibrosis and inflammation and favor healing processes.[28]

Similarly, fat injection aimed at improving scars most likely brings improvement through mesenchymal cells and numerous growth factors already contained in the lipoaspirate, which contribute to skin and scar remodeling. In patients with scars that were treated by this technique, one of the main related improvements was the increase in elasticity and malleability of the scar tissue. This could be partially caused by the marked increase in the number of elastic fibers, easily perceived microscopically in postinjection scar samples, in consequence of these injections. This improvement could be related to the number of injections and/or the time elapsed postinjection (**Fig. 18**).[29,30]

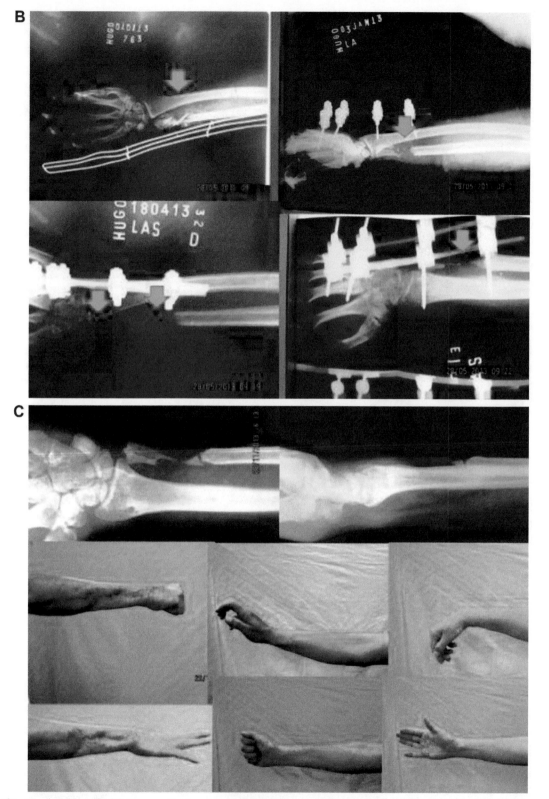

Fig. 14. (*continued*). (*B*) Same patient, original (*top left*) and follow-up radiographs after bone debridement elsewhere (*top right*) after three fat injections at fracture site, with new bone formation at 4 (*bottom left*) and 5 months (*bottom right*).Top left arrow shows fracture site, *top right arrow* shows missing bone site. *Lower left arrows* show shade of new bone formation. *Lower right arrow* show new bone formation. (*C*) Same patient at 8 months, after four injections (two injections after healing at 3-month intervals): bone connecting at ulnar void site (*top left*), with minimal dorsal deviation (*top right*); results at 8 months with no hypertrophy, no tendon adhesions, and practically normal function (*middle and bottom*).

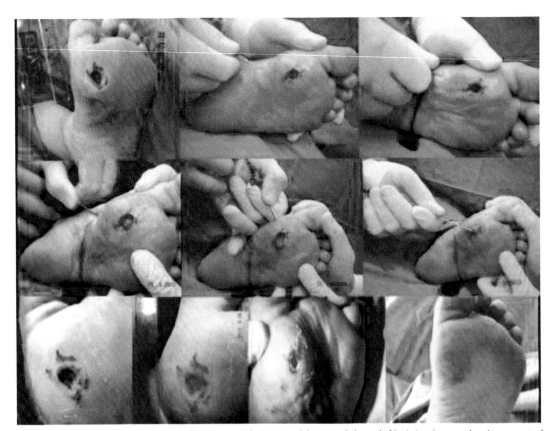

Fig. 15. A 43-year-old woman with diabetes with 2-year-old wound (*top left*); injection under (*top center*), around (*top right*, *middle left*, *center*), and in the wound (*middle right*); at 2 days (*bottom far left*); 4 days (*bottom left*); 11 days (*bottom right*), and at 8 months (*bottom far right*). Wound was healed in 42 days. No hypertrophic scarring, practically normal appearance.

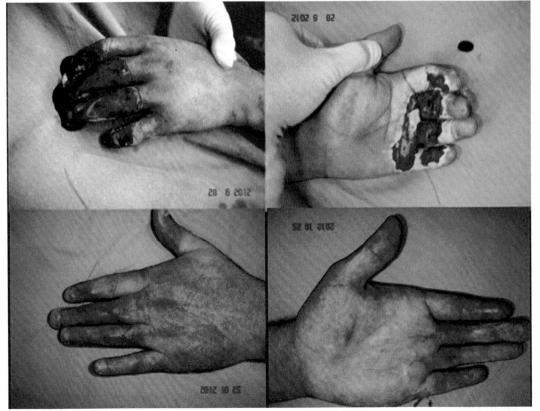

Fig. 16. A 22-year-old patient burnt on clothes ironing press; treated with debridement and one fat injection under all areas of the wound; 8 weeks after healing, with no hypertrophic scarring and practically normal skin.

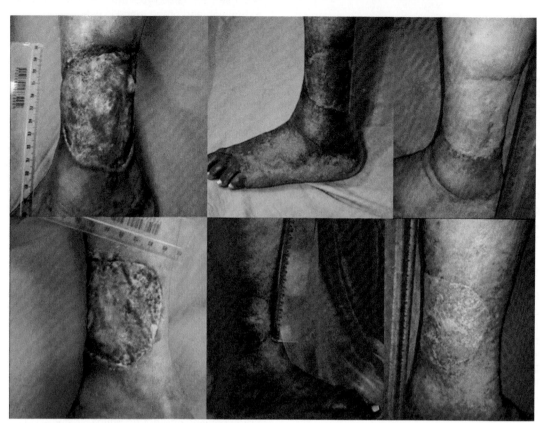

Fig. 17. Original aspect of 7.5-year-old venous ulcer (*left*); 3 months postcure (*center*); 7 months postcure (*right*). No hypertrophic scarring (same patient in **Fig. 7**).

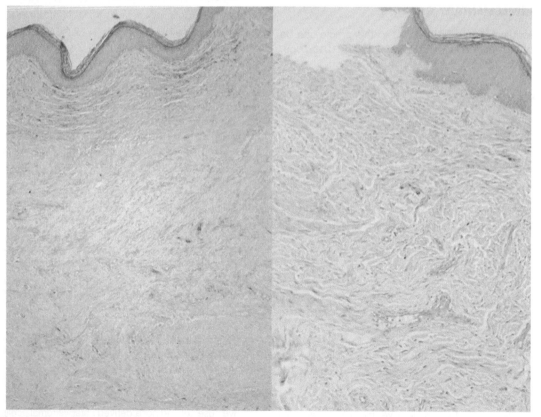

Fig. 18. Microphotograph of a biopsy of preinjection hypertrophic scar tissue (*left*) and of scar tissue on the same site (*right*) 3 months after the injection (Vierhoff staining, original magnification ×100) demonstrating a large amount of small elastic fibers (*in black*) intermingled within the collagen fibers network.

There are many publications in the literature where authors indicate that the method of harvesting and the way that the lipoaspirate is handled, enriched, or injected could influence the result of each one specific fat injection procedure. We believe that the Coleman technique provides a standardized method with a very short learning curve for the surgeon and with an easy-to-learn routine for the entire surgical team. Procedures practiced and results presented by different surgeons will make these results easier to compare when the harvesting and preparation of the fat is done with a similar technique or method.[31–34]

SUMMARY

Fat grafting as an adjuvant treatment of burn and other wounds favors healing, while decreasing the usual healing time and fostering lesser to practically no hypertrophic scarring. When used under scars or immediately over joint spaces it diminishes fibrosis, diminishing scar thickness and allowing for more pliability of the skin and for recovery of the joint normal spaces. It may also favor bone formation aiding in bone fractures and segmental bone loss recovery.

SUPPLEMENTARY DATA

Supplementary data related to this article can be found online at http://dx.doi.org/10.1016/j.cps.2014.12.009.

REFERENCES

1. Zuk PA, Zhu M, Mizuno H, et al. Multilineage cells from human adipose tissue: implications for cell based therapies. Tissue Eng 2001;7:211–28.
2. Zhu M, Ashjian P, De Ugarte DA, et al. Human adipose tissue is a source of multipotent stem cells. Mol Biol Cell 2002;13:4279–95.
3. Fujimura J, Ogawa R, Mizuno H, et al. Neural differentiation of adipose-derived stem cells isolated from GFP transgenic mice. Biochem Biophys Res Commun 2005;333(1):116–21.
4. Dominici M, LeBlanc K, Mueller E, et al. Minimal criteria for defining multipotent mesenchymal stromal cells, the International Society for Cellular Therapy position statement. Cytotherapy 2006;8:315–7.
5. Rigotti G, Marchi A, Galiè M, et al. Clinical treatment of radiotherapy tissue damage by lipoaspirate transplant: a healing process mediated by adipose derived adult stem cells. Plast Reconstr Surg 2007;119:1409–22.
6. Gimble JM, Katz AJ, Foster SJ. Adipose-derived stem cells for regenerative medicine. Circ Res 2007;100:1249–60.
7. Akita S, Akino K, Hirano A, et al. Non-cultured autologous adipose-derived stem cells therapy for chronic radiation injury. Stem Cells Int 2010;2010: 532704.
8. Brown SA, Levi B, Lequeux C, et al. Basic science review on adipose tissue for clinicians. Plast Reconstr Surg 2010;126:1936–46.
9. Coleman SR. The technique of periorbital lipoinfiltration. Operat Tech Plast Reconstr Surg 1994;1:120–6.
10. Coleman SR. Long term survival of fat transplants: controlled demonstrations. Aesthetic Plast Surg 1995;19:421–5.
11. Coleman SR. Structural fat grafts: the ideal filler? Clin Plast Surg 2001;28:111–9.
12. Coleman SR, editor. Structural fat grafting. St Louis (MO): Quality Medical Publishing; 2004.
13. Kim W, Park BS, Sung JH, et al. Wound healing effect of adipose-derived stem cells: a critical role of secretory factors on human dermal fibroblasts. J Dermatol Sci 2007;48:15–24.
14. Lolli P, Malleo G, Rigotti G. Treatment of chronic anal fissures and associated stenosis by autologous adipose tissue transplant: a pilot study. Dis Colon Rectum 2010;53:460–6.
15. Bene MD, Pozzi MR, Rovati L, et al. Autologous fat grafting for scleroderma-induced digital ulcers. An effective technique in patients with systemic sclerosis. Handchir Mikrochir Plast Chir 2014;46: 242–7.
16. Klinger M, Marazzi M, Vigo D, et al. Fat Injection for cases of severe burn outcomes: a new perspective of scar remodling and reduction. Aesthetic Plast Surg 2008;32:465–9.
17. Viard R, Bouguila J, Voulliaume D, et al. La lipostructure dans les sequelles de brulures facials. Ann Chir Plast Esthet 2012;57:217–29.
18. Sultan SM, Barr JS, Butala P, et al. Fat grafting accelerates revascularization and decreases fibrosis following thermal injury. J Plast Reconstr Aesthet Surg 2012;65:219–27.
19. Carpaneda CA, Ribeiro MT. Study of histologic alterations and viability of adipose grafts in humans. Aesthetic Plast Surg 1993;17:43–7.
20. Carpaneda CA, Ribeiro MT. Percentage of graft viability versus injected volume in adipose autotransplants. Aesthetic Plast Surg 1994;18:17–9.
21. Klinger M, Caviggioli F, Klinger F, et al. Autologous fat graft in scar treatment. J Craniofac Surg 2013; 24:1610–5.
22. Matsumoto D, Sato K, Gonda K, et al. Cell-assisted lipotransfer: supportive use of human adipose-derived cells for soft tissue augmentation with lipoinjection. Tissue Eng 2006;12:3375–82.
23. Yoshimura K, Sato K, Aoi N, et al. Cell assisted lipotransfer for cosmetic breast augmentation: supportive use of adipose-derived stem/stromal cells. Aesthetic Plast Surg 2008;32:48–55.

24. Yoshimura K, Sato K, Aoi N, et al. Cell-assisted lipo-transfer for facial lipoatrophy: efficacy of clinical use of adipose-derived stem cells. Dermatol Surg 2008; 34:1178–85.

25. Eto H, Suga H, Matsumoto D, et al. Characterization of structure and cellular components of aspirated and excised adipose tissue. Plast Reconstr Surg 2009;124:1087–97.

26. Gentile P, De Angelis B, Pasin M, et al. Adipose-derived stromal vascular fraction cells and platelet-rich plasma: basic and clinical evaluation for cell-based therapies in patients with scars on the face. J Craniofac Surg 2014;25:267–72.

27. Liao HT, Marra KG, Rubin P. Application of platelet-rich plasma and platelet-rich fibrin in fat grafting: basic science and literature review. Tissue Eng Part B Rev 2014;20:267–76.

28. Sultan SM, Stern CS, Allen RJ Jr, et al. Human fat grafting alleviates radiation skin damage in a mu-rine model. Plast Reconstr Surg 2011;128:363–70.

29. Bruno A, Santi DG, Fasciani L, et al. Burn scar lipo-filling: immunohistochemical and clinical outcomes. J Craniofac Surg 2013;24:1806–14.

30. Pallua N, Baroncini A, Alharbi Z, et al. Improvement of facial scar appearance and microcirculation by autologous lipofilling. J Plast Reconstr Aesthet Surg 2014;67:1033–7.

31. Jauffret JL, Champsau P, Robaglia-Schlupp A, et al. Playdoyer en faveur de la greffe adipocytaire de S.R. Coleman. Ann Chir Plast Esthet 2001;46: 31–8.

32. Herold C, Pflaum M, Utz P, et al. Vitalitätsvergleich von fetttransplantaten welche mit der coleman tech-nik und dem tissue trans system (shippert methode) gewonnen wurden. Handchir Mikrochir Plast Chir 2011;43:361–7.

33. Nguyen PS, Desouches C, Ga AM, et al. Develop-ment of micro-injection as an innovative autologous fat graft technique: the use of adipose tissue as dermal filler. J Plast Reconstr Aesthet Surg 2012; 65:1692–9.

34. Fisher C, Grahovac TL, Schafer ME, et al. Com-parison of harvest and processing techniques for fat grafting and adipose stem cell isolation. Plast Reconstr Surg 2013;132:351–61.

Index

Note: Page numbers of article titles are in **boldface** type.

A

Adipocytes, in grafted fat, conclusive schema for, 187, 188

Adipogenesis/regeneration process, 186, 187, 188

Adipose-derived stem cells, and adipose tissue, cryopreservation of, **209–218**
   cryopreservation of, 213–215
      recommended protocol for, 215
   for fat grafts, 206
   therapy based on, and autologous fat grafting, for tissue construction after cryopreservation, 216
   transfer of, may replace transfer of adipose tissue, 214–215

Adipose-derived stem/stromal cells, condensation of, by reduction of adipocytes and tissue volume, 193–194
      by supplementing stromal vascular fraction, 194
      for therapeutic use, 196
   importance of, in grafted tissue, for adipose regeneration after fat grafting, 192

Adipose stem cells, **169–179**
   adipogenic differentiation of, 171–172
   and bone marrow-derived stem cells, 171, 172
   and tumor cells, interactions between, 173–174
   biology of, 181–182
   isolation and characterization of, 169–173
   regenerative potential of, 174–175
   regulation of, 174
   to enhance fat grafting, 173

Adipose stromal/stem cells, 156
   cell surface markers for, 156, 157
   chondrogenic differentiation in, 158
   differentiation of, into skeletal muscle cells, 158–159
   ectodermal differentiation of, 159
   immunomodulatory effects of, 159
   secretion of cytokines and growth factors by, 159–160
   tumorigenesis and, 161–163

Adipose tissue, and adipose-derived stem cells, cryopreservation of, **209–218**
   and stem/progenitor cells, **155–167**
   as cell source, for development of cell-based therapies, 161
   as source of cells for tissue engineering, 156
   confocal microscopy of, 171
   cryopreservation of, 212–213
      as variable in fat processing, 210
   importance of, 209–210
      recommended protocol for, 214
   injury to, 183–184
   intact, and aspirated fat tissue, difference between, 192
   ischemia to, 182–183
   liposuction harvested, 156
   mechanical force of, 184–185
   structure of, 182, 183
   transfer of, may replace transfer of adipose-derived stem cells, 214–215

B

Brazilian buttock technique, **253–261**

Buccal area, fat grafting in, 235–236

Burns, and wound healing, 263–264
   burn scars, and difficult wounds, fat grafting for treatment of, **263–283**

Buttock augmentation, aesthetic considerations for, 254–255
   fat grafting for, history and evolution of, 253

C

Cell-based regenerative medicine, regulation of, 162–163

Cheek, fat grafting in, 228, 229

Chin, fat grafting in, 228–231

Cryobiology, fundamental, cryopreservation processes and, 210–212

Cryopreservation, of adipose-derived stem cells, 213–215
      recommended protocol for, 215
   of adipose tissue, and adipose-derived stem cells, **209–218**
      as variable in fat processing, 210
      future perspectives in, 215–216
      importance of, 209–210
      recommended protocol for, 214
   of fat cells, process, injury mechanisms, work for, 211
   of whole fat tissue, 211–212
   tissue construction after, autologous fat grafting, and adipose-derived stem cells-based therapy for, 216

Cryopreservation processes, fundamental cryobiology and, 210–212

Cryoprotective agents, addition to and removal of, from fat cells, 210–211

Clin Plastic Surg 42 (2015) 285–287
http://dx.doi.org/10.1016/S0094-1298(15)00010-3

Printed and bound by CPI Group (UK) Ltd, Croydon, CR0 4YY

03/10/2024

01040382-0009